Twelve Steps for Those Afflicted With Chronic Pain

Twelve Steps For Those Afflicted With Chronic Pain:

A Guide to Recovery from Emotional and Spiritual Suffering

Stephen Colameco M.D., M.Ed., F.A.S.A.M.
Redington Shores, Florida

For my wife, Sheran,
and our children—Jennifer, Andréa
David, Marie and Christopher

Twelve Steps for Those Afflicted With Chronic Pain

Second Revised Edition 2013

Copyright 2005 © Stephen Colameco M.D., M.Ed.

TABLE OF CONTENTS

ACKNOWLEDGMENTS

The author would like to thank Gina Lovrencevi for her editorial assistance. The author is grateful to Drs. Seddon Savage and Mark Scheutzow who encouraged him to update and revise the first edition of this book. .

.

Preface (First Edition)

Modern medicine has made remarkable advances, perhaps none as important as the development of powerful painkillers and surgical anesthesia. Today, we take these once revolutionary innovations for granted but without them, physicians would be unable to relieve pain in those with illness, injury, or in need of surgery. Relieving pain and suffering has always been a fundamental obligation for all physicians. Having made progress in treating pain caused by acute illness, injury, and medical procedures, researchers have turned their attention to the problem of chronic pain.

In the last decade of the twentieth century, pain management emerged as a specialty, and it is not surprising that anesthesiologists were among the first physicians to train in the treatment of chronic pain. Simultaneously, magnetic resonance imaging (MRI) became widely available, allowing physicians to see inside the human body in ways they could never do before; whereas x-ray images only show abnormalities in bone, MRI provides physicians with detailed images of soft tissues, such as muscle, nerves, and cartilage. MRI allows pain specialists to see abnormalities that might cause chronic pain and guided by these images, they are able to inject medications into difficult to reach areas such as the spine.

When pain management procedures are not successful, physicians can often turn to newer, more powerful painkillers.

Pharmaceutical companies responded to a growing need for chronic pain medications with products such as OxyContin®, Duragesic®, and Opana®. For many, modern medicine offered hope that pain could be eliminated. However, for most, the reality is that modern medicine can afford only partial relief for their suffering.

For many individuals, chronic pain is a not a condition that can be cured as much as managed. In most cases, successful management requires more than drugs and medical procedures in most cases. Chronic pain is now universally recognized as a complex biopsychosocial condition. All too often, physicians and their patients seek only to treat "medical" causes for chronic pain, relying exclusively on medications and procedures while overlooking the importance of more integrated, comprehensive treatment approaches.

I am an addiction specialist. Most physicians have little interest in treating addicts, let alone addicts who complain that they are in pain and need stronger medications. Sadly, chronic pain is very common among addicts. Managing chronic pain in addicts is more complicated than treating acute pain. It requires an understanding of both addiction medicine and of pain management. There have been very few controlled medical research studies specifically addressing the problem of pain management in patients with addiction. Studies published in medical journals mostly deal with the use of new pharmaceutical treatments, and drug companies do not usually recruit addicts for pain research. Psychology and social work publications emphasize the importance of behavioral treatments for addiction and pain, but they do not address the many complicated medical issues. In order to be a complete addiction specialist, I had to learn more about pain management, particularly about the psychological and social factors that contributed to my patients' suffering. I needed to learn how to manage chronic pain in patients at increased risk for addiction without making matters worse.

Treating addicts with pain poses special problems. On the one hand, patients have a right to expect that doctors will treat their pain. On the other hand, physicians do not want to make the problem of addiction worse by prescribing opioids to addicts. Addressing acute pain in an addict is usually a straightforward problem for an addiction specialist. Acute pain can and should be managed, but addicts often need more medication than others do. As an example, a heroin addict might come to the hospital for a serious infection caused by a dirty needle. Since he is used to injecting large amounts of heroin every day, he might need ten times the amount of morphine than most to relieve his pain. Most doctors and nurses are uncomfortable with administering high doses of opioids to any patient, let alone a known addict. They are concerned that addicts might want more medication just to get high—or worse—that prescribing high doses of medication might lead to overdose at the hospital.

As the only addiction specialist in a busy community hospital, I spent a good deal of time educating hospital staff about the treatment of pain in patients with a history of addiction. The hospital where I worked appointed me to its pain management committee and asked me to attend medical staff meetings where I educated physicians about the importance of adjusting pain treatment to fit individual patient needs. Board-certified pain specialists at the hospital concentrated their efforts on treating pain with interventions such as spinal injections, but they did not provide hospital consultations for chronic pain management. I found myself serving as a general pain management consultant, who provided care for all patients, including those with addiction problems. Almost all of these patients had previously seen family physicians, orthopedic and pain specialists, but continued to suffer from chronic pain. Most of these patients not only suffered from physical pain, but also from emotional and spiritual pain. For two years, I worked as a member of the hospital inpatient psychiatric team. Many of the psychiatric patients whom we treated had chronic pain and addiction problems. This experience confirmed my belief that emotions play a powerful role in a patient's pain, and that behavioral treatments were needed to complement traditional medical care.

The healthcare industry divides care treatment into separate medical, psychiatric, and addiction components. Modern neuroscience teaches us that psychiatric and addictive disorders are brain diseases, often treatable with medications, but medications are not the only way to change brain chemistry. Brain imaging studies have shown that meditation, prayer, and psychotherapy can also change brain chemistry. The artificial division of healthcare into medical, psychiatric, and addiction treatment services only makes sense as a relic from a time when medical problems were considered physical, psychiatric problems considered mental, and addiction problems considered moral or behavioral problems. The structure of the healthcare delivery system makes it difficult to treat chronic pain when accompanied by addiction or emotional distress. Addiction treatment centers may not accept patients who are being treated for chronic pain and many pain specialists will not treat addicts or those with serious psychiatric disorders. The lives of those who suffer from untreated, chronic pain quickly spiral out of control, and those afflicted often become desperate for help. They might frequent hospital emergency departments, doctor shop, or turn to the street in order to get pain medications. Without proper treatment, their emotional and physical suffering intensifies.

As I struggled to find better ways to help my patients, I found that I had to look beyond medical research studies. A review of the psychology and social work literature led me to believe that recovery from chronic pain has many parallels to recovery from addiction. The majority of chronic pain patients I treated were in need of recovery from the effects of pain on their lives. Many were in need of recovery from childhood emotional trauma. The medical system had failed them, and, in some cases, had actually contributed to their suffering as a result of ill-advised medical treatments, or by convincing them that the cause of their suffering was solely physical injury or illness.

The treatment of chronic pain with medications sometimes parallels the treatment of addiction and other psychiatric disorders. There is no single treatment that can eliminate chronic pain, because chronic pain is a complex experience with many causes. There is no single treatment for emotional suffering, because it too has many causes. It stands to reason, then, that medications are never the single treatment for chronic pain, just as they are never the single treatment for emotional illness. Medications alone rarely cause the alcoholic to stop drinking, the anxious to stop worrying, or the depressed to overcome negative thinking. Medications are an important part of the treatment for chronic pain and emotional disorders, but not the sole treatment.

When doctors concentrate their treatment solely on the physical aspects of chronic pain, they enable patients just as doctors who deal solely with the physical aspects of alcoholism enable alcoholics. Many doctors are unwitting enablers of alcoholics. They treat consequences of alcoholism such as trauma, liver, nervous system, pancreas, or cardiac complications—failing to adequately address the underlying cause: alcoholism. Doctors enable chronic pain patients when they ignore emotional and social factors that contribute to pain. As an example, pain specialists often assume that bulging spinal discs apparent on MRI are the cause of a patient's chronic back pain and recommend injection treatments to reduce inflammation. While these treatments may help acute flare ups, there is little scientific evidence supporting the benefit of such treatments for chronic back pain. This should not be surprising, since most adults with bulging spinal discs do not have chronic back pain. When physicians fail to recognize and address emotional or spiritual suffering that contributes to chronic back pain, they become enablers.

Pain patients routinely come to my office carrying their MRI pictures and medical records, telling me that they had seen many specialists, tried injections, nerve stimulators, and opioid medications. They come to my office assuming that medical treatments had failed because theirs were particularly difficult cases. They come to my office in desperation, hoping a different doctor and a different medication might help. They are often angry, resentful, and depressed. As often as not, their family life is in shambles. They are usually surprised when I begin asking questions about their mood, emotional development, and spiritual beliefs. Desperate for help, they put up with my questions. Like alcoholics powerless over the effects of alcohol, these individuals are powerless over the fact that they have pain. In recovery, alcoholics learn to accept what life brings, live one day at a time, and to recognize their limitations. My patients learn that they couldn't change the past or the fact that they have a painful medical condition. They learn to accept what life brings, to live one day at a time, and to recognize their inability to control situations.

The medical approach to chronic pain usually defines successful treatment as reduced pain. At each visit, doctors ask patients about their pain—typically using a 1-10 scale. When patients report lower pain scale scores after starting a new medication, the treatment is deemed successful. Unfortunately, the medical approach rarely leads to elimination of pain, and often fails to improve overall well-being and function. The

Twelve Step approach to chronic pain does not promise elimination of pain. It offers hope for emotional growth, spiritual growth, and improvement in social function. This approach requires self-assessment and commitment to personal growth no matter what the starting point. Any patient with chronic pain can benefit from participation, regardless of pain severity or disability.

I wrote this book in the tradition of using the Twelve Steps to serve a population in need of recovery. There have been many programs built upon the Twelve Step foundation of Alcoholics Anonymous, including Al-Anon, Narcotics Anonymous, Adult Children of Alcoholics, Cocaine Anonymous, Emotions Anonymous, and Overeaters Anonymous. Individuals with chronic pain may have found recovery by participating in one or more of these programs. However, other suffering from chronic pain had no reason to attend any of these programs. They need to recognize that their emotional and spiritual suffering contributed to their pain. They need to learn a better way to cope. In short, they needed a Twelve Step recovery program that deals specifically with the effects of pain on their lives.

This book borrows from the teachings, traditions, sayings, and prayers of AA. In some instances, I have modified well-known sayings and writings to specifically address the needs of those afflicted with chronic pain. I am indebted to all of those individuals who have contributed to the recovery tradition. It is my sincere hope that those who follow these Steps will organize groups in their own communities. Recovery is for all of us.

Introduction

Pain is a uniquely individual experience; it changes from moment to moment. Pain is difficult to describe in words. Factors such as body position, mood, distraction, and atmospheric conditions can change the amount of pain or how it feels. This intensely personal nature of pain complicates scientific research, making it more difficult to study than other medical conditions. As an example, it is much easier for researchers to measure the effects of a new blood pressure medication because scientists have agreed on standard ways to measure blood pressure. Scientists studying the effects of a new pain medication are left with subjective measurements that often change throughout the day. Difficulty in measuring pain is one of the many reasons that physicians are unsure about treatment effectiveness.

The earliest attempts to explain the mechanisms of pain were based on pain sensation thresholds and bodily injury models. These were the simplest types of pain to study. These experiments often involved applying increasing pressure or heat to the skin of volunteers. Researchers could measure when subjects felt pain and/or how much heat they could tolerate. Scientists have also studied how the body responds to different types of injuries. Research into the body's reaction to physical injury has taught us a great deal about inflammation, pain pathways, stress hormone release, blood vessel changes, nervous system responses, the cognitive experience of pain, and much more. However, these types of research did little to explain why some individuals suffer from chronic pain in the complete absence of any detectable physical injury, or long after acute injuries have healed.

Since theories about pain based solely on bodily injury models could not completely explain chronic pain, researchers turned their attention to psychological causes. Psychologists and psychiatrists emphasized the importance of emotional difficulties and what they call "secondary gain motivation," such as the prospect of receiving a large disability payment. However, the psychological models failed to explain why individuals without significant emotional difficulties developed chronic pain. Today, researchers are working on integrative theoretical models to better explain the nature of chronic pain. Integrative approaches are better suited to explaining conditions with many components and contributing factors, such as physical conditions, personality, heredity, prior pain experiences, pain-related beliefs, spirituality, and psychological states.

The perplexing interaction of pain and emotions begins at birth. An expectant woman in active labor experiences significant pain during womb muscle contractions. Her pain may be influenced by expectations about birthing, emotional support of loved ones, worries about her child, and many other factors. Her newborn infant announces passage from the comfort of the womb to the outside world with anguished cries. Why does he cry? Is he experiencing physical discomfort caused by change in temperature, sight, and sound? Or is he suffering a devastating emotional trauma as primal scream therapists would have us believe? Whatever the reasons, it is clear to all of those in the birthing room that the infant is distressed and needs emotional comforting. Upon first seeing her crying infant, the mother may cry as well, but hers are not tears of pain. Rather, the pain of labor is mixed with her overwhelming joy. Physical pain and emotions dynamically interact with each other in both mother and newborn.

As children grow older, they learn to control how they react to pain. Whether they are hurting emotionally or physically, they are often taught to express their pain in words and to hold their back tears. By the time children reach puberty, society expects that they will no longer cry when they experience physical pain. Perhaps this is the reason that many cultures mark the passage from childhood into adulthood with special rites that demand courage in the face of pain. Participants in rites of passage must endure painful experiences, such as body piercing, circumcision, or multi-day survival tests. After completing such ritual tests, adolescents are accepted into society as young adults. Having learned their lessons, young adults try not to show emotional or physical pain. They learn to maintain control over their negative feelings. Societies do make exceptions when it is acceptable for adults to cry in public—notably in times of great sorrow and grief, such as at funerals.

Most people are fortunate enough to live without thinking about pain except when beset by acute injury or illness. For them, pain has a purpose. Acute pain lets them know their bodies need attention, whether in the form of an aspirin, or visit to the doctor. Chronic pain is an altogether different matter. Chronic pain seems purposeless. Chronic pain is disabling because it takes away the ability to perform activities that others consider routine. Those with chronic pain are often irritable, angry, depressed and overly dependent on others. They are left wondering why they are in pain when others are not, what they might have done to deserve this fate.

If healthcare providers are to treat chronic pain effectively, they must address more than bodily injury. They must also concern themselves with patients' emotional distress and spiritual conflicts—because these too contribute to suffering. The medical community and the public became increasing aware of the problem of untreated chronic pain in the 1980's and 1990's. Physicians, mostly anesthesia and physical medicine specialists, sub-specialized in the newly created specialty of pain management. These specialists learned how to perform procedures such as spinal injections and nerve blocks to relieve painful conditions. The United States Congress designated 2000 to 2010 as the "Decade of Pain Control and Research." With the increasing concern about chronic pain came an increased willingness of physicians to prescribe opioid medications, especially the newer formulations such as OxyContin®, Duragesic® and Opana®.

Have the efforts of physicians and pharmaceutical companies reduced the burden of pain-related suffering and disability? One would hope so, but there is very little data showing that new technologies actually improved patient well-being and reduced disability costs. [1][2][3] Despite the wide-spread acceptance of medical treatments among physicians, there remains little clinical evidence supporting effectiveness in treating many chronic pain conditions. Comprehensive reviews published in major medical journals concluded that there is no proven long-term benefit to spinal injection treatments for chronic low back pain, yet, physicians increasingly perform these procedures. [4][5][6][7] Research also questions the value of opioid medications for the treatment of certain types of pain. Although physicians prescribe opioids to treat fibromyalgia—a painful condition affecting about 3% of adult women, this practice is not supported by the scientific literature.[8] Also, newer, more expensive medications, such as OxyContin ® may be no better than older opioid formulations.[9] Furthermore, opioid medications may not improve mood or social behavior in chronic pain patients.[10] Over time, opioids in high doses may actually heighten sensitivity to pain, so the brain may start interpreting normal sensations as painful. The term for this is "hyperalgesia". In such cases, pain decreases when opioids are tapered.

Medical treatments are usually based on the bodily injury model of understanding chronic pain, failing to consider the psychological, social, and spiritual factors. Most chronic pain patients have been seen by physicians who based evaluation and treatment solely on the bodily injury rather than an integrative model. Physicians typically approach chronic pain in the same manner as they would approach other medical problems. When evaluating a patient with chronic pain, physicians develop a "differential diagnosis" or a list of possible causes for the pain. They narrow this list through the use of diagnostic studies in order to find an anatomical or physiological problem that might be causing the pain. As an example, when patients present with chest pain, physicians immediately consider the most serious possibilities, such as heart attack, lung collapse, blood clots in the lungs, pneumonia, etc. and narrow the list by gathering more information through the use of diagnostic tests such as EKGs, stress tests, and x-rays. Physicians evaluating patients with chronic back or neck pain typically place high value on the importance of Magnetic Resonance Imaging (MRI) studies, because plain x-rays do not show herniated discs or nerve compression. When physicians find an abnormality on MRI that might explain back pain, they are apt to believe that they have found the principal cause, however abnormal MRI findings such as disc bulges and arthritis are very common among patients without back pain.[11][12] This is not to say that MRI is of no value as a diagnostic tool; rather MRI testing is greatly overvalued by physicians and patients alike. In one study, MRI results affected treatment in only 6% of cases.[13] Similar results have lead experts to conclude that MRI scanning may be no better than plain x-rays.[14][15][16][17] All too often, patients bring their MRI films to a new doctor as proof that MRI abnormalities show the sole cause of their pain. In reality, pain is a complex phenomenon in which biological (e.g. disc bulges), social (e.g. social support, employment) and psychological (e.g. anger, depression, anxiety) factors dynamically interact with one another. Modern medicine treats the biological problems associated with chronic back pain with spinal injections, nerve stimulators, nerve blocks, manipulation, physical therapy, anti-inflammatory, anti-seizure and opioid-type medications. Despite good intentions, medicine rarely cures chronic pain, so patients must learn to accept some degree of pain, even with the daily use of strong opioid medications. For many patients, the medical system, bolstered by its marketing and advertising, creates the false hope that pain can be adequately treated by addressing biological factors alone.

Moreover, emphasizing pills and procedures often delays effective treatment for psychological factors that contribute to suffering, while fostering what has been called the Chronic Pain Syndrome or "sick role". Psychological, social, and spiritual concerns should be addressed as soon as possible without unduly emphasizing one aspect of care over another. Scientific researchers agree that there is a strong link between chronic physical pain and emotional problems. [18 19 20 21 22 23 24 25 26]

In many cases, a psychological assessment can predict response to treatment when an MRI cannot. [27] Chronic pain patients are more likely than others to have had emotional difficulties before seeking medical care; such difficulties include depression, anxiety, alcoholism, drug abuse, or having been abused as children. [28 29 30 31 32 33 34 35]

Physicians have a duty to relieve pain and suffering. They also have a duty to minimize harmful treatments. From ancient times, physicians have used derivatives of the poppy plant to treat pain. Today, naturally occurring medications, such as morphine, remain among the most widely prescribed of all medications because they effectively treat severe, acute pain. Chronic pain has always been more difficult to treat than acute pain, and physicians have long recognized that physical dependence or frank addiction can complicate treatment. Despite these risks, opioids remain as important a treatment option today as they were 1000 years ago. In recent years, the pharmaceutical industry has developed more potent synthetic opioids and improved delivery systems such as time-released pills and skin patches. Although opioids remain a mainstay of chronic pain treatment, they seldom provide the answer because they treat only one component of pain. The question for most patients is rarely, "Am I in pain?" but more often, "How much pain can I tolerate?" Sometimes, these medications do more than deaden pain; they also numb feelings and emotional pain. Some individuals feel energized and less fearful when they take these medications, so they begin to use their prescribed opioids to deal with fatigue or anxiety. Opioids are wonderful painkillers, but they are not an effective treatment for emotional problems that so often accompany pain: depression, fear, anxiety, guilt, worry, or anger. Numbing feelings with medications only delays getting the type of real help that might relieve emotional suffering. Even worse, it might lead to addiction.

While it is true that many people have benefited from the physicians' increased willingness to prescribe opioids for chronic pain, there has been an unintended negative consequence; increased availability of prescription opioids has helped spread an epidemic of drug abuse and dependence, especially among young adults. The National Survey on Drug Use and Health (US) documents the rapid rise in prescription drug use for non-medical reasons. In 2010, more than 12 million people reported using prescription opioids either, without a prescription or for reasons other than for pain relief.[36]

Many patients who suffer from addiction also have chronic pain, a fact that complicates treatment for either condition. One might think that addicts treated with methadone—a powerful opioid—would experience very little chronic pain, but the opposite is true. About one-third of patients on methadone treatment for addiction suffer severe, chronic pain of over six months in duration, and almost half believed their pain actually led to their addiction.[37] [38] All patients deserve pain relief, including addicts but treatment with opioids alone often fails. For many patients the untreated part of chronic pain is the emotional suffering that contributes to their pain experience. Methadone does little to treat depression, anxiety, or Post-Traumatic Stress Disorder!

If modern medicine is not the answer, what hope is there? Hope lies in the distinction between pain and suffering and in understanding the role emotions play in the pain cycle.

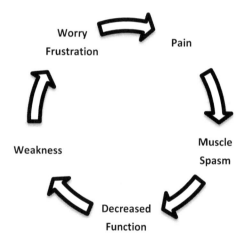

Modern medicine can reduce pain, but it rarely addresses the worry and frustration that are part of the pain cycle. Patients with chronic pain may be powerless over the fact that they have pain in their lives, but they are *not* powerless over how they deal with pain. There is a growing body of scientific evidence supporting behavioral approaches to pain management.[39][40] The Cochrane Library of Systemic Reviews, an authoritative source of information regarding clinical evidence, has not found sufficient evidence to support spinal injections for chronic back pain, however it has found research support for cognitive behavioral therapies and interdisciplinary care.[41][42]

Fibromyalgia is a pain condition that is often vexing for patients and physicians; although there are FDA approved medications to treat this condition, reviews of the scientific literature have concluded that this condition often responds to non-pharmacological treatments.[43][44] This is not to say that chronic pain patients should avoid medications or procedures. Research on injection treatments and medications may be inconclusive because they fail to identify those patients least likely to respond, (i.e. those with emotional suffering). Also, psychiatric medications can treat many emotional difficulties, such as anxiety, depression, or insomnia. Patients who continue to suffer after failing medical treatment with opioids, psychiatric medications, and procedures often become desperate and sometimes try unproven or dangerous treatments. Before resorting to such treatments, patients should consider proven behavioral approaches.

Twelve Step programs of recovery may offer a unique solution for individuals suffering from chronic pain conditions. There was a time when the medical profession was skeptical about Twelve Step programs because these programs were "non-professional" and because researchers found it difficult to study a program that stressed anonymity. Today, medicine accepts the value of the twelve steps as a "standard" part of addiction treatment, and contemporary research seeks to learn why Twelve Step programs work and which types of clients are most likely to benefit from participation.[45][46][47] All Twelve Step programs emphasize overcoming negative behavior such as isolation, blame, resentment, obsessive worry, compulsive self-reliance, inappropriate dependency and self-pity. These are the same problems that so often afflict chronic pain patients.

The aim of Twelve Step programs is to help clients overcome negative beliefs, negative behaviors, and self-centeredness through active participation in these programs. For Twelve Step programs that help individuals stop using drugs or alcohol (e.g. AA) sobriety is considered a necessary first step in recovery. The desire to stop drinking or using drugs is not a precondition for participating in other Twelve Step programs (e.g. Al-Anon). What binds the diverse 12-Step programs together is not sobriety, but recovery. Recovery requires a commitment to active participation in a program of emotional and spiritual growth. Many psychologists would argue that Twelve Step programs are effective because they use cognitive behavioral therapy (CBT) techniques. Cognitive Behavioral Therapy is effective for the treatment of depression, anxiety, panic disorder, phobias, and other conditions—often just as effective as medications. Of course, AA began almost a half-century before CBT became widely accepted. The fact remains that individuals who actively "work" Twelve Steps programs change their beliefs about themselves, their beliefs about others, and their behaviors. In the process, they improve self-esteem, relationships, social function, and conscious contact with a Higher Power.

The twelve steps presented in this book are intended to help individuals recover from the emotional suffering that so often accompanies chronic pain. Just as participation in AA does not preclude pharmacological treatment with antidepressant medications or Antabuse®, participation in this program does not preclude medical treatments. Addiction specialists know that medications alone rarely lead to sobriety, let alone recovery. They know that recovery often requires both medical and behavioral treatments. This program draws upon the rich tradition of other Twelve Step programs and of cognitive behavioral therapy. For those who have failed traditional medical treatments, such as medications, surgery, and spinal injections, these steps offer hope for a better future with little, if any, risk. They offer a solution to problems that contribute to pain suffering, (e.g. lack of trust, fear, worry, blame, isolation, and resentment). They provide a path for recovery from suffering—a path that leads to trust, honesty, reconciliation, peace and joy.

12 Steps for Chronic Pain

1. Admitted that we are powerless over our pain—that our lives had become unmanageable.

2. Came to believe that a Power greater than ourselves could help us find strength in our adversity and fulfillment in our lives.

3. Made a decision to turn over our will and our lives over to our Higher Power.

4. Made a searching and fearless morale inventor of ourselves.

5. Admitted to our Higher Power, to ourselves, and to another human being the exact nature of our wrong.

6. Were entirely ready to have our Higher Power remove all these defects of character.

7. Humbly asked our Higher Power for the strength to overcome our shortcomings, so that we can carry out the Higher Power's will for us.

8. Made a list of all the persons we had harmed because we were controlled by our pain and our fear, and became willing to make amends to them all.

9. Made direct amends to such people wherever possible, except when to do so would injure them or others.

10. Continued to take a personal inventory of our strengths and our weaknesses, and promptly admit when we harm others or ourselves.

11. Sought through prayer and meditation to improve our conscious contact with our Higher Power, praying only for knowledge of our Higher Power's will for us and for the power to carry that out.

12. Having had a spiritual awakening as a result of these steps, we sought to carry this message to others and to practice these principles in all of our affairs.

Chapter 1

Old Ways of Coping No Longer Work

Chronic Pain Step 1: Admitted that we are powerless over our pain—that our lives had become unmanageable.

Marie's Story

"I could not believe my life was turning out the way it was. I had done everything I could to make my family proud. We grew up poor, and Mom worked two jobs. I helped out with my brothers and sisters. When other children in the neighborhood were getting in trouble, I stayed home and studied. We lived in a rough neighborhood, and I was one of the lucky ones who went to college. I earned a degree in nursing and went to work in a hospital ICU. I married a wonderful man, moved to the suburbs, and began raising a family. A few years later, I hurt my back. My pain has gotten worse and worse. I had MRI tests and saw pain specialists. I began to miss work because of pain. I found myself worrying more and more. I hardly ever got a good night's sleep because of pain and worry. Over time, I began to live from pain pill to pain pill, finding little real relief. Soon I was taking more medicine than prescribed. My life was out of control…"

Our Lives have Become Unmanageable

We suffer from chronic pain. We have sought relief from family doctors, orthopedist surgeons, chiropractors, physical therapists, and pain specialists. We have tried medications, manipulation, injection treatments, and surgery to relieve our pain. We may have tried copper bracelets, magnets, hypnosis, and other unconventional methods. Sometimes, these treatments helped, at least for a while, but we are still in pain. Because of our pain, we are no longer able to perform our normal activities. Many of us have had to interrupt our careers and have suffered financially. Some of us no longer enjoy exercise, dining out, sexual activity, social functions, or playing with our children. We are often irritable, and "short" with our friends and family. Our lives have become unmanageable.

We Cannot Change the Fact of our Pain

Everyone experiences illness and physical injury at some time in their life. Everyone experiences pain and discomfort—some more than others. As we age, our bodies begin to deteriorate and we lose the ability to do things we once enjoyed. None of this is personal. It is not a form of punishment. Medical science may be able to extend life and relieve pain, but it will never be able to change the fact that we age and experience pain. Pain is part of the universal experience of humankind—a fact we cannot change.

It is Time to Try a New Way to Deal with Pain

Despite all of our efforts and the efforts of healthcare professionals, we still suffer. Our way of dealing with pain has not worked, and it is time to try a new way. We may be filled with negative thoughts about our predicament. We may have had angry thoughts about how we were injured or how others treated us. We may have thought about our injuries over and over again—only adding to our distress. Or we may have thought about how pain has kept us from doing the things we wanted to do. Perhaps we worried about what other people might think of us, so we avoided situations where others might see our limitations. We might have gone from one doctor to another, hoping the next would be better or smarter than the last. Whatever we have tried in the past, it no longer seems to work. Negative thinking has kept us trapped in the past. It is time to try a new way of dealing with our pain.

Pain is Unique to Each of Us

Modern science has taught us a great deal about pain. We know that there are different types of pain. Some pain is due to acute injury. When someone with a sprained ankle tries to run, she will immediately experience a sharp pain that tells her to stop and rest the ankle. Inflammation causes specific types of pain receptors in the ankle to send signals along fast nerve fibers to the spinal cord and then to the brain. Because ankle sprains result in stretching and tearing of ligaments, we initially treat them with anti-inflammatory medications, ice, and rest. When the inflammation subsides, so does the pain. The pain caused by diabetic nerve injury is an entirely different type of pain with a different cause. People who have diabetic nerve damage (i.e. diabetic neuropathy) usually describe pain as burning. Unlike the acute pain of an ankle sprain, this type of pain travels along slower nerve fibers, and there is no swelling, redness, or other signs of inflammation, so ice and anti-inflammatory medications are of little value. It is difficult to treat this type of pain, but it does respond to anti-seizure or antidepressant medications. Many patients with back ailments have a mixture of local inflammation pain similar to that of a sprained ankle, muscle spasm, and spinal nerve irritation.

For all that modern science has learned about pain, there is far more yet to be discovered. Why do some people seem to have a high pain threshold—like those who can have dental cavities filled without any medication? Why so many older adults are hunched over from spinal fractures, degenerated discs and arthritis yet have no serious pain? Why do others with only a few bulging spinal discs have severe pain? The simple truth is that each of us experiences pain differently, and that many factors influence when and how we experience pain. Emotions are one of these factors.

Our Emotions and Our Pain

Most of us recognize the powerful role that emotions play in our experience of pain. We have all heard stories about soldiers injured in battle, only realizing they had been wounded when someone notices blood on their uniforms, or of football players finishing a game with what appeared to be an ankle sprain, only to learn later that the injury was a fracture. The soldiers and football players who do not notice serious injuries are usually so "pumped" with adrenaline that they stay focused on the job at hand. They are distracted from their injuries.

When a child falls and bruises his knee, his mother often "kisses away" the pain. It may seem silly to adults, but children stop crying soon after Mother applies the healing kiss and says, "There now, all better." The positive feelings associated with love and caring are often enough to treat the child's hurt.

Most of us have had tension headaches from time to time, and we understand that emotional stress causes this type of headache. Doctors usually call them stress or muscle contraction headaches. We readily accept the fact that worry, time pressure, and other hassles can cause and aggravate headaches. We also know that relaxation, distraction, massage, and painkillers all make it better. But painkillers alone can mask the underlying problem: stress. If we do not deal with the stress, the headache will return with a vengeance when the painkiller wears off. And taking more painkillers will make the problem worse. Ignoring the stress often leads to more frequent and more severe headaches.

Stress, worries, and concerns not only cause pain, they also change the way we experience pain. Consider how our perceptions can change how we might experience common heartburn. We have all seen or read advertisements for heartburn or acid reflux disease treatments. Most of the time, we recognize it for what it is—irritation of the esophagus caused by reflux of stomach contents. Usually, we won't give it much thought, but might take a heartburn remedy, such as Maalox ®, Pepcid ®, Prilosec ® or Zantac ®. However, if we had just learned that our younger brother had had a heart attack, we are likely to experience this same heartburn very differently; the pain might be much more intense, shoot into our throat or down our arm. Our concern might cause our esophagus to go into spasm. We might call 911 instead of dismissing the pain as heartburn. Our worries, concerns, and our health beliefs affect how we perceive pain and how our body reacts to painful stimuli.

There are good reasons for emotions and pain to be linked. The pain-emotion connection plays an important role in the survival of all animals. If our pet dog, Fido, runs across a porcupine and ends up with a few needle sticks, he learns an important lesson. Fido forms a pain memory associated with porcupines. Fido may not understand a porcupine in exactly the same way we might, but seeing or smelling a porcupine is all that is necessary to trigger the pain memory in Fido. Upon seeing or smelling this prickly animal, his brain signals release of stress hormones, such as adrenaline and cortisone. Fido's heart and breathing rates rise. His blood vessels constrict. His blood sugar level rises and his blood supply shifts from internal organs to his leg muscles so that he can run away— FAST. Fido also exhibits signs of what we might call fear, with bristling hair and tail between his legs, he scurries away from the porcupine. Painful memories and stress hormone release are linked in all animals. What happens to Fido also happens to us humans!

We can also learn about the mind-body connection by studying language. There are many expressions that describe how the body reacts to emotions. If we are really stressed, we may tell a friend that we are "uptight." Our friend might tell us to "hang loose." Most of us understand that "uptight" and "hang loose" refer to parts of the human anatomy. If we tell a friend that we were frightened by something that happened, we might say that this event "scared the s _ _ t out of me." If we lose the affection of someone dear to us, we say we are heartbroken and actually feel this grief in our chests. Emotions, especially fear, anger, and grief, have a strong effect on how we experience pain.

Stress Adds to Our Pain

In our society, we tend to lump all of our negative feelings into one term—stress. If we are having a bad day, we say that we are stressed or stressing. Though it is difficult to actually define what we mean by stress, we share some common understanding that we are running on emotional overload.

When we are relaxed and interested in our work, we are often so engrossed in our activities that we pay little attention to our bodily feelings. Time passes quickly and we may not be at all aware of our aches and pains. But when we are stressed, we experience pain quite differently, as shown in the two scenarios that follow:

Scenario 1:

Marge met her good friend Sandy at a restaurant for lunch. They had not seen each other in weeks, and were enjoying each other's company. While chewing her food, Marge felt a sharp pain and realized she had cracked a tooth. Startled, she said to Sandy, "I think I cracked a tooth. I'll have to try to get in to see the dentist later today."

Scenario II:

Marge met her good friend Sandy at a restaurant for lunch. They had not seen each other in a few weeks. Marge had just learned that her husband had been having an affair and he wanted a divorce. She was distraught, angry with her husband, and frightened about her future. She hardly ate a thing. While chewing her food, she felt a sharp pain and realized she had cracked a tooth. Wincing, she said, "I can't believe it. I think I cracked tooth. What else can go wrong? I think I'd better leave."

When we are overloaded with worry, anger, hate, fear, or shame, we experience pain differently. Because negative feelings are themselves emotionally painful, they intensify physical pain. In the two scenarios above, Marge cracked the same tooth while eating the same food in the same restaurant with the same friend. The nerve endings around her cracked tooth signaled her brain that something was wrong with the tooth—a signal she interpreted as pain. In the first scenario, her brain was receiving pain signals from her tooth as well as positive feelings from her brain's emotion centers. In the second scenario, Marge's brain had to process two painful experiences at the same time. As a result, she experienced the pain of the cracked tooth more intensely than in the first scenario.

Psychologists have long recognized the important role emotions play in pain. In 1970's the Canadian psychologist Ronald Melzack began collecting "pain words" and placing them into categories that ultimately became the McGill Pain Questionnaire that is widely used in pain centers today; the questionnaire asks patients to choose words from a list that best describe their pain. The McGill Pain Questionnaire provides information about pain intensity, character and emotional response. Researchers now turn to modern technologies to better understand the relationship between emotions and pain. They are conducting controlled experiments using functional magnetic imaging (fMRI) scans to measure brain activity in response to painful stimuli and the effects of negative emotions such as anxiety and fear. Chronic pain is a disease of the central nervous system, affected by many factors including our emotions.

Medications May Numb Our Feelings

Many of the medications used to treat chronic pain are central nervous system depressants or have abuse potential. Alcohol is one of the oldest medications used to treat pain. Alcohol was once used widely in "patent medications" and elixirs, but most alcohol use for pain management today is self-medication. Alcohol is a central nervous system depressant. While many find that it relieves pain and may induce sleep, over time it tends to increase pain by disrupting normal sleep, causing depression and may lead to alcohol abuse or dependence. Physicians do not prescribe alcohol for pain management, but they do prescribe other medications that affect the same brain binding sites (GABA receptors) as alcohol and have many of the same risks including dependence and withdrawal. These medications include certain muscle relaxants, sleeping pills and anti-anxiety medications. While they may seem to work in the short run, studies show that patients consuming these medications are at risk for poor outcomes—lower functional levels, drug abuse, and unintentional overdoses. They are often prescribed along with opioids.

Of all the medications used to treat chronic pain, no class of medications has received more attention than opioids. Opioids (also known as opiates or narcotics) include codeine, morphine, oxycodone, buprenorphine, hydrocodone and others. They attach to specific binding sites called opioid receptors located in many parts of the body—especially the spinal cord and the brain. Opioids have many effects on the body, including reducing pain, suppressing cough, narrowing pupils, sedation, decreasing the breathing "drive" and causing constipation. These drugs also affect emotions. For some individuals, opioids reduce anxiety in social situations. Others find that these drugs are exhilarating and give them energy. For many, they numb negative feelings and make them forget about their worries. However, over time, it takes more and more medication to achieve these effects—a condition we call "tolerance." Once individuals develop a tolerance, stopping opioids suddenly usually results in withdrawal symptoms such as sweats, anxiety, muscle aches, nausea and diarrhea.

Though many of us need medications to relieve our pain, we must always be watchful for signs of increasing emotional distress. When pain is well controlled with medications, our lives should be better. We should be less concerned with our own problems and more actively involved in the lives of those around us. If our lives have become increasingly unmanageable, we must consider whether the improper use of medications may be contributing to our misery.

Many of us have never abused drugs or alcohol in the past, so we might find it difficult to believe that we are having a problem now. We need to carefully consider our emotional state at the time we first began consuming these medications on an ongoing basis. If we had an injury or a surgical procedure, did we need to remain on medication longer than our doctors anticipated? Did our pain continue long after our wounds healed? If so, is it possible that we were using medications for something other than their ability to relieve the pain of physical injury? Were we under a lot of stress at the time? Were we fearful of pain and take medication before physical therapy sessions? Did we continue using them because they helped us relax, gave us energy, or numbed emotional pain? If so, we need to talk with our doctors about changing our treatment plans.

We Have only One Life

We humans have an amazing capacity to deceive ourselves. Most of us go about our daily routine as if we were going to live for a very long time. We make plans for the future, not considering the fact that we might not live long enough for these plans to matter. Of course, we know we have only one life and that death is inevitable, but we push these thoughts to the extreme recesses of our minds. Because we might live to a ripe old age, planning makes sense. Compared to other creatures on this planet, we have incredible brain power to solve complex problems, but this also comes at a cost. Life planning would be much simpler if all we needed to do were to build a nest and bury chestnuts to prepare for winter. We must plan for education, careers, weddings, retirement, and the needs of future generations. Our ability to think and plan is what makes us human, but this same intelligence also gives us an immense capacity to fool ourselves. We spend far too much time thinking about the past—something we cannot change. We spend far too much time planning for the future—something we cannot control. We must learn to live "one day at a time." Worry just adds to our distress, so it is time to stop dwelling on our past and stop wasting our energy trying to control the future.

Inspirational Reading—Helen Keller

"Although the world is full of suffering, it is full also of the overcoming of it."

"Character cannot be developed in ease and quiet. Only through experience of trial and suffering can the soul be strengthened, ambition inspired, and success achieved."

"Many persons have a wrong idea of what constitutes true happiness. It is not attained through self-gratification, but through fidelity to a worthy purpose."

"Security is mostly a superstition. It does not exist in nature, nor do the children of men as a whole experience it. Avoiding

danger is no safer in the long run than outright exposure. Life is either a daring adventure, or nothing."

Can you imagine being a two-year-old girl who could neither see nor hear? Can you imagine the physical pain that must come from constantly falling and bumping into things? Or the emotional pain that comes from not being able to tell your mother that you are hungry, cold, tired, or hurting? Can you imagine the isolation such a girl would have experienced?

When Helen Keller was a year old, she became ill and lost both her vision and hearing. Her parents knew that Helen needed help, but did not know where to turn. When Helen was seven years old, they hired a tutor named Anne Sullivan.

Anne was a remarkable woman in her own right—intelligent, intuitive, and energetic. Since it had been so difficult for Helen's parents to communicate limits and rules, Anne had to be strict with Helen. But Anne's discipline was matched by an indomitable spirit, so she would not accept failure as an option. Within a few days of becoming Helen's tutor, Anne had taught Helen how to spell words with her hands, but Helen did not understand what the words meant! One morning Anne spelled "W-A-T-E-R" into one of Helen's hands while she placed the other hand into a stream of water coming from a pump. This was the breakthrough that changed both Helen's and Anne's lives. The feeling of water running over Helen's hand turned the letters of the word in the other hand into something that had real meaning. Immediately, Helen bent down and tapped the ground; Anne spelled "E-A-R-T-H." Helen understood!

When Helen was ten years old, Anne began teaching her how to speak. She did this by spelling words, and then saying them while Helen held a hand over Anne's mouth. Often people could not understand what Helen was saying, but she did not give up. With time, she learned to be understood.

Helen learned to recognize Braille characters with her fingers. Once she learned Braille, she could then read books. Helen did not stop at reading Braille versions of English books. She also learned to read French, German, Greek, and Latin! At age 20, she entered Radcliff College. From 1946 to 1957, Helen traveled around the world, visiting 39 countries and speaking about her experiences and advocating for the rights of people who are deaf or blind. Her book, *The Story of My Life*, has been translated into 50 languages.

There is much we can learn from the life of Helen Keller. She was powerless over the fact that she was deaf, dumb, and blind, but with the help of Anne Sullivan, she was able to overcome seemingly insurmountable problems posed by these conditions. We too are powerless over the fact that we have painful medical conditions, but we, like Helen Keller, can overcome seemingly insurmountable problems. Many of us need a breakthrough, as when Anne held one of Helen's hands under the running pump water and spelled the word "water" in her other hand. We cannot be content with accepting our lots in life, as Helen's parents were not content to accept Helen as an unruly, handicapped child. We must seek others who are dedicated to helping us, and learn to trust them. Above all, we must learn that we are powerless without the help of others and without the help of a Higher Power in our lives.

Prayer for the First Step

I admit that I am powerless over the fact that I have pain. I admit that my life has become unmanageable and that suffering has taken over my life. Help me understand that I can no longer manage on my own. I am ready for help.

Exercise for the First Step

This exercise helps us recognize that our lives have become unmanageable. We must honestly answer each of the following questions in detail:

-Do you often feel like giving up because you can't make things better?

-Do you find that medication has become the center of your life, and that you live "pill to pill"?

-Does it seem like there is little hope that you will find real satisfaction in the future?

-Do you have trouble dealing with difficulties that others seem to handle without becoming upset or "stressed"?

-Are you worried that you will be too dependent on others?

If you answered yes to most of these questions, then your life has become unmanageable. You may already recognize that you are not able to handle the problems that life presents. You probably do not feel optimistic about your future, and may not believe you have the power to improve your life. If you accept the fact that your old ways are no longer working, and that your life is now unmanageable, then you are ready to move on to the next step.

Chapter 2

Accepting the Higher Power's Role in our Recovery

Chronic Pain Step 2: Came to believe that a Power greater than ourselves could help us find strength in our adversity and fulfillment in our lives.

Peter's Story

"My family doctor sent me to a pain specialist because I needed a lot of pain medication. I had already been to other specialists and had injections into my lower back. I expected the same type of questions from the new doctor as the others had asked me, but this is not at all what happened. He wanted to know the story of my life…

My father was a preacher, but he also had to work a regular job. My mother had a rough life; her father had been an alcoholic. She had her hands full working and raising the family. My mother was not the warm, affectionate type. My two brothers got in trouble in school and later became alcoholics. I tried really hard to be good… to make my Mom and Dad proud. I was a shy child, and I stuttered when I was young. As a teenager, I overcame my shyness and became a popular athlete. After serving in the Army, I became a respected law enforcement officer— until I injured my back at work and had to go out on disability. I go to church every Sunday. I don't gamble, swear, drink, or cheat. Why did God punish me with this horrible pain?

After listening to my story, the doctor told me that going to church every Sunday is not the same as spirituality, and that I needed to ask for God's help in order to deal with my suffering. He told me that spirituality was not as much about not doing bad things as it was about doing the right things. He told me that God puts obstacles in our path for a reason. My back injury was one of those obstacles."

Accepting the Higher Power's Role in our Recovery

Spirituality can be defined in many ways, but most would agree that a spiritual life is one where there is a sense of purpose and a feeling of connectedness to something greater than oneself. Throughout the ages, many people have found religious practice as important to their spiritual growth. However, for some of us, negative experience with organized religion may have caused us to reject the entire notion of spirituality. Some of us were raised without religion in our lives. Others may have had negative experiences. Some were brought up in overly strict households where fear of damnation was more important than love; others may have been physically or sexually abused by clergy. For these and other reasons, we may be suspicious of Twelve Step programs because they emphasize the importance of belief in a Higher Power. All too often, we confuse religious belief and practice with spirituality.

Religious beliefs and practices have changed greatly over the centuries. As societies have changed, religions have had to change their teachings and practices to reflect the new attitudes and beliefs of their membership. As an example, Christians no longer hold to teachings that the sun revolves around the earth, that slavery was ordained by God, or that clergy should torture accused witches into confession—yet these beliefs were once supported by the Christian Church. Religious practices continue to evolve. As they have throughout history, most young people adopt the religion of their parents. Because the political, educational, economic, social, and scientific institutions of society affect what people believe, with each passing generation religious norms change. In the past half-century, women have increasingly entered occupations that had been previously the exclusive province of men. As society has come to accept women in their new roles, religions have had to reevaluate the traditional belief that only men could serve as clergy. Today, most Christian denominations accept women ministers and liberal churches have moved on to debate more controversial topics such as whether practicing homosexuals should be ordained.

Churches, mosques, synagogues, and temples are sacred places where many of us choose to join together in worship. Twelve Step meetings are also sacred places because we come to these rooms for understanding, fellowship, and prayer. What binds us together is not the place where we pray, but the fact that we come together seeking a closer connection with a Higher Power and to find real purpose in our lives. Many people choose not to attend Twelve Step meetings because they are skeptical of the spiritual basis of the program. In most cases, such objections are a cover-up for the real reason—fear.

It has been said that all evil in the world can be traced to fear. It has also been said that all goodness in the world comes from love. Fear is the power that keeps us apart from one another. Love is the power that brings us together. Each of us harbors fear. Each of us struggles to overcome fear. Every great reformer had to overcome his or her fears—fear of criticism, shunning, or even torture and death. Each great reformer took personal risk. Each followed the will of a Higher Power. Those who are skeptical of spirituality should learn from the lives of the many courageous men and women who chose love over fear. It was through their efforts and personal sacrifices that the world has become a better place. We owe our freedoms to these men and women, and to the higher purpose that guided their lives. Were it not for their efforts, we would still live in a society that allowed slavery, torture, child labor, and oppression of women. Many of the great reformers were guided by strong spiritual convictions. And for each courageous leader, there had to be legions of willing followers who also dedicated their lives to a higher purpose.

There are those who say that there cannot possibly be a Higher Power because a loving God would never allow suffering on earth. They might condemn the notion of a Higher Power because they are afflicted with chronic pain. They are wrong. They fail to understand that the Higher Power works within history, not apart from it. They fail to understand that each of us has a part to play in making creation a better place. They fail to understand that their criticisms of others' beliefs may be a manifestation of fear—a way to stay apart from others rather than seeking common ground. We need not be afraid to join our Twelve Step fellowship, because we welcome into our program anyone who seeks recovery from chronic pain.

Many among us are agnostic or atheists who do not believe in God and this can be obstacle to getting started in a Twelve Step program. According to the Big Book of Alcoholics Anonymous (AA), about half of the original AA fellowship was agnostic or atheist and the challenge became to develop a fellowship that would be inclusive of religious and nonreligious members. The Big Book chapter entitled "We

Agnostics" lists alternative concepts (i.e. Creative Intelligence, Spirit of the Universe, Love, God of Reason, Great Reality) to a traditional God. Some agnostics conceptualize a Higher Power as an inner wisdom or higher self that guides them. Some consider the Higher Power as a Unity: the interconnected web of existence of which we are a part. It is said that the Buddha compared being afflicted with bodily pain to being struck by an arrow and the mental suffering (e.g. self-pity, anger, resentment, depression, fear) that often accompanies bodily pain as like being struck by a second arrow; the wiser person stops with the first arrow. Meditation, an essential part of Buddhist practice, has now become a pain management treatment offered in many interdisciplinary pain programs. By practicing meditation, agnostics may be able to reduce suffering while at the same time developing a personal spiritual practice. Agnostics who choose to follow the twelve steps have many ways of conceptualizing a Higher Power.

Each of us needs forgiveness. Each of us needs understanding. Each of us needs purpose in our lives. Each of us needs spirituality. The twelve steps are a spiritual journey that complements religious practice. For some of us, the twelve steps enrich our religious experience. For others the twelve steps are a way to find spirituality outside of organized religion. As they say in AA: "It works if you work it."

We Can Change How Pain Affects Our Lives

Many of us have become depressed, anxious, or ashamed because of our pain or disability. We may have isolated ourselves from those who love us. We may have been consumed by anger and bitterness. Some of us may have lost our spiritual focus, or even have become angry with the Higher Power. We cannot change the fact that we have pain, but we can develop a healthy, positive attitude toward life. Emotional suffering is not the inevitable result of physical illness. It is the optional part of our pain experience. We may always have some degree of physical pain and limitation, but we do not have to be depressed, fearful, or bitter. Pain can be a "wake up" call for us to look at our lives and make needed changes. Maybe our lives were not so great before our pain began. Maybe we were already suffering emotionally because of unresolved childhood trauma such as physical or sexual abuse. Many of us were depressed or overly fearful as children. We may have come from homes where we did not receive the love or security we needed. We may be living in unfulfilling or abusive relationships. We may have been on the brink of despair when our painful medical conditions pushed us over the edge. We can continue living life the same way. Or we can learn new, healthier ways of coping.

We need to be honest with ourselves. Were we really happy and fulfilled before we developed a painful medical condition? Do we really want to go back to the way things were? Or do we want to change, to learn from our pain, and become more whole? We come together with a feeling of hope, knowing that others have recovered from the affects of chronic pain, are no longer controlled by their suffering, and have learned to live whole and healthy lives despite physical problems.

Pain—Our Motivation to Change

Why is there suffering in the world? Is there any meaning or purpose to our existence? Few people believe that life is a random, purposeless, material existence. If there is purpose in life, then there must also be meaning in our suffering.

Civilization's earliest written documents ask the same question we ask: "Why is there suffering in the world?" Suffering is a central theme of the *Bible*. In the Book of Job we learn about a good and pious Job who suffers great misfortune and physical pain. Job enters into a dialog with God wherein he asks why the wicked prosper while the just suffer. Chastised by God, Job is humbled and repents his requests for justice. Biblical scholars debate the meaning of God's "speeches" in the Book of Job. Some interpret these speeches as a repudiation of human's right to question God. Others interpret them as telling us that humans are incapable of understanding the nature of the universe, so we cannot explain why a righteous man should suffer. Like Job, we are left to find meaning in our own lives and in suffering.

Finding Meaning in Our Lives

Many of us have stumbled through life with no sense of purpose. When we were children, we played with our toys and dreamed of growing up to become fire fighters, fashion designers, engineers, nurses, or, perhaps, even action heroes! Finding meaning in life was hardly a question when we were young. Somewhere along the path from childhood into adulthood, we may have lost our way. We probably have asked ourselves, "Is there more to life than this?" Perhaps we thought meaning would come through marriage and a good job, but many of us found ourselves in troubled marriages or unfulfilling careers. In order to find real meaning in our lives, we need a connection to something greater than ourselves. We need spirituality. We need the presence of a Higher Power in our lives.

Hope

Our acceptance of our powerlessness over pain leads us to look outside of ourselves for answers. The Second Step is often called the Hope Step. We should be comforted by the fact that millions of people have come to the Second Step and millions of individuals have benefited from active participation in other 12-Step programs. In order to recover, they had to give up their compulsive self-reliance and place hope in the Higher Power. We too must overcome our fears and learn to hope. What choice do we really have?

Inspirational Reading—A Hymn by John Newton

Amazing grace! How sweet the sound That saved a wretch like me. I once was lost, but now am found, Was blind, but now I see.

'Twas grace that taught my heart to fear, And grace my fears relieved. How precious did that grace appear The hour I first believed.

Through many dangers, toils and snares I have already come; 'Tis grace hath brought me safe thus far And grace will lead me home.

The Lord has promis'd good to me, His word my hope secures; He will my shield and portion be, As long as life endures

Yes, when this flesh and heart shall fail, And mortal life shall cease; I shall possess, within the vail, A life of joy and peace.

The earth shall soon dissolve like snow, The sun forbear to shine; But God, who call'd me here below, Will be forever mine.

In the eighteenth century, the British navy could force teenage boys to serve aboard their warships. John Newton began his sailing career when he was involuntarily pressed into service. Life aboard a sailing ship was difficult, and the punishments for breaking rules were harsh. He tried to escape, but he was caught and suffered the consequences: public whipping. Shortly afterwards, he was forced to become a servant on a slave ship. The shipmaster was very cruel and brutally beat John on several occasions. He again escaped, but this time he was not caught. John Newton continued working as a seaman—the only job he knew. He worked hard and was promoted to the rank of captain. He was the master of his own ship, but on a ship with an unfortunate mission: delivering slaves to the Americas.

While attempting to navigate through a violent storm off the coast of Africa in May 1748, John Newton prayed to God for deliverance. That night his prayers were answered. He survived the storm and in the process had a spiritual awakening. He committed himself to follow the will of the Higher Power, even though that meant leaving the security and income that came from being a captain.

In later years, John Newton became a minister. In 1772, he wrote a poem for his congregation to show how grace had helped him survive his turbulent seafaring days, ultimately carrying him from the high seas to the church pulpit. His poem became the lyrics to one of the most beloved of all hymns: "Amazing Grace." This hymn has been an inspiration to countless people, especially those who have had to endure difficult, painful times. "Amazing Grace" is one of the most widely recorded hymns, with popular artists introducing the hymn to succeeding generations of listeners, many of whom had never heard it sung in a church.

The truth of this hymn is universal. That is, each of us must deal with our own "trials, toils, and snares." In order to find peace, we each must overcome our fears, and learn to accept whatever life hands us. John Newton faced difficult times, and

23

he also did wretched things, but if he had not been aboard a slave ship on that stormy night in 1748, he might never have had his spiritual awakening.

The Higher Power works in mysterious ways. John Newton transported Africans in chains to America. The descendants of those very slaves adopted Christianity, and they found strength in words written by a man who at one time was the captain of a slave ship! "Amazing Grace" teaches that there is meaning in suffering. It teaches us that the Higher Power works in real time, through the efforts of individual men and women. Even as we sail through turbulent seas of chronic pain, we can move forward with our lives, contributing greatly to the lives of others.

Prayer for the Second Step

I pray for an open mind and open heart so I can come to believe in a Power greater than myself. I am suffering and I know I need help.

Exercise for the Second Step

For some of us the concept of a Higher Power is difficult to accept. This exercise helps us escape from our isolation and learn how the Higher Power works in the real world.

Religious scholars and philosophers use the word "transcendent" to describe the Higher Power. To "transcend" means to go beyond or surpass the limits of ordinary power. We come to know of the presence of the Higher Power in our lives by identifying those experiences that carry us beyond the ordinary limits of our lives.

In the coming weeks, make an effort to listen to music, watch movies, read books, call friends, and, perhaps, visit places that are special to you. If you attend a church, mosque, synagogue, or temple, begin your week with a day of worship. In this exercise, we look for signs that the Higher Power is working in our lives.

Music:

Music has been called the universal language. It can transcend national boundaries. It eradicates our worries and move us to a better place. Music therapy helps patients with chronic pain, headaches, and other medical problems. Even though they might not understand the German lyrics, just listening to Beethoven's "Ode to Joy" brings many people to tears. For others, hearing "Amazing Grace" evokes a strong, positive emotional response. Music can play an important role in our recovery.

Are there hymns, songs, or other forms of music that distract you from your pain and move you to a better emotional and spiritual place? List them.

Plan to listen to music that has special meaning for you during the coming week. If you listen to talk radio while you commute to work, turn it off and listen to music instead. If you find that you daydream or worry while listening to music, sing along with the music! It is difficult to daydream while singing! Notice how music helps you become less aware of your pain.

Sacred places:

Are there places that have special meaning for you, places that inspire a sense of awe or where you feel a sense of connection to nature? For some, sacred places are churches, mosques, synagogues, or temples. Ancient religions designated special places in nature where they believed their gods dwelt—a sacred grove of trees for example. When we visit sacred places our thoughts become less cluttered, and we become aware of the presence of the Higher Power in our lives.

List those places that are important for you. What makes them so special?

If you can, visit one of these places in the coming weeks. Notice whether you are more in touch with your feelings, or whether you feel more connected to other people when you visit your sacred place. Notice if your pain is less when you are there.

Special people:

Have you noticed that you are more at ease in the presence of some people, and more nervous or anxious around others? Have you noticed that some people seem to be more accepting of you and less likely to find fault? Have you noticed that you want to confide in some people but not others? These are special people in your life. They can play a positive role in your recovery.

List the special people in your life. Why are these people different from others?

Make a point of either spending time with them, or call them on the telephone. Notice if your pain decreases when you are around them.

Movies and Television:

The media has transformed society. For many of us, movies and television connect us with something greater than ourselves. They can stir our emotions and motivate us to become better people.

List the films or television shows that most deeply moved you, and explain why.

Choose one film that most stirs your emotions. Plan to watch it one day this week. When you watch your special movie, be aware of your emotional reactions. Did the film bring up feelings that you have been ignoring? If you watched the movie with a friend, how did this affect your experience?

Books:

Books can be powerful forces in our lives. Unlike movies that we usually watch from beginning to end, we rarely finish a book at one sitting. Usually, we set the book aside, giving us time to digest what we have read. When we were young, our teachers made us read biographies of famous people. These assignments were intended to inspire and teach us the value of dedication and hard work. Books have played an important role in changing society. The sacred texts of religious faiths— the *Bible, Qur'an*, *Upanishads*, *Book of Mormon* and many others have played a huge role in shaping society as we know it, and continue to be among the most read books today. Works of fiction can also influence society. Harriet Beecher Stowe's novel *Uncle Tom's Cabin* was published in 1852 and helped turn the tide of American opinion against slavery. A few years later, Charles Darwin published what many believe to be the most influential scientific work ever written: *On the Origin of Species by Means of Natural Selection, or The Preservation of Favored Races in the Struggle for Life*. Prior to Darwin, most scientists never considered the fact that species might come and go. Darwin's theories forced religious thinkers to consider new ways of understanding traditional creation teachings. Books continue to influence how we think and what we believe. Books may have had an important role in shaping your beliefs. Rereading the books that most affected your life might help you on your road to recovery.

27

List the books that most affected your life and explain why.

Are there lessons in these books that still apply today? Do you still find inspiration in them?

Chapter 3

We Do Not Have to Suffer Alone

Chronic Pain Step 3: Made a decision to turn over our will and our lives over to our Higher Power.

Faith's Story

"I have suffered with chronic pain throughout most of my life. It began with pain in my lower abdomen when I was a teenager. I have had so many operations that it is hard to count, and the operations caused adhesions—scar tissue that binds my intestines and causes even more pain. It was during one of my hospitalizations when my surgeon called in an addiction specialist to see me. Everyone believed I was addicted to opioids. My name was listed in the hospital emergency department as a known addict. As I lay in my hospital bed needing IV medications every two hours, I was beginning to wonder myself!

The addiction specialist told me I was what they call a 'pseudo-addict.' I had unrelieved chronic pain. My pain was real. I shared with him something I had not told doctors before—that I had been sexually assaulted as a child. Until now I had never dealt with my emotional pain.

It has been three years since I began my recovery. I still have episodes of bowel obstruction, but I go to the hospital much less than before. I have learned to share my feelings with those I trust. I am active at my church. I pray every day and thank God for my blessings. Nowadays, I spend less time alone and more time with family and friends. I have even been able to return to part-time work. I have learned that emotional suffering adds to physical pain and that I needed more than just medication."

We Do Not Have to Suffer

Pain and suffering are not the same. Pain is best a considered as a physical sensation. Scientists can measure pain thresholds through experiments such as applying increasing amounts of pressure to peoples' arms to determine precisely how much pressure is needed before they feel pain. People have different pain thresholds for different types of pain. As an example, some people can tolerate having dental cavities filled with little or no local anesthesia, but these same individuals might not be able to tolerate eating jalapeño peppers. We all experience pain differently. Suffering is a state of ill-being, hopelessness, or misery that often accompanies pain. We can learn new ways of coping that serve to alleviate our suffering.

Isolation and Suffering

When we are in pain, we often isolate ourselves from friends and family. When we isolate, we put ourselves in our own personal prison—a prison called self-absorption or self-centeredness. We become prisoners in solitary confinement, and we are our own jailors! Each moment we spend lamenting our own situation is time that could be better spent engaged in the lives of others.

"Who? Me? Self-absorbed? No way!" When we first consider this possibility, we react with disbelief, saying to ourselves, "Of course I am always thinking about myself. You would too if you were in chronic pain!" But the more we consider the facts, the more we come to realize that our isolation and negative thinking contribute greatly to our suffering.

The bars on our prison cells are not made of steel, but made of distrust, fear, bitterness, compulsive self-reliance, compulsive worry, and resentment. Since we are the wardens of our own personal prisons, we have a choice. We can stay in prison or we can use the keys of the Twelve Steps to open the doors and set ourselves free.

We know that some inmates are more comfortable inside the prison walls than outside. They have become accustomed to living in this way. Despite all of its restrictions, prison seems safer to these folks than freedom. Experts tell us that this is one of the reasons why many parolees commit crimes shortly after their release. On the outside, parolees face challenges they did not face in prison. They must find employment, deal with coworkers, and reconnect with family and friend. Many parolees find these challenges overwhelming, so they turn again to a life of crime or drugs.

Like prisoners in real jail cells, there are many reasons why we might want to stay behind the bars we have created for ourselves. We might be afraid to trust people, so we won't let ourselves form meaningful relationships. We might be afraid of failure, so we don't risk taking chances. We might criticize others' actions, convincing ourselves that our way is the only right way to do things. In the process, we cut ourselves off from life's opportunities. We cut ourselves off from other

31

people and the support they can provide for us. When we are unaware that we have created our own personal prison cell, we are in denial.

Denial is a powerful force that keeps us from seeing the truth about our lives. Each of us has our own history, and each of us has many reasons for avoiding painful facts about our lives. If we are to move forward with our recovery, we must own up to the past. We must allow ourselves to feel the pain of sadness and grief. Overcoming denial is essential to recovery. No matter how hard we try to convince ourselves otherwise, the simple truth is that none of us can live without the help of other people. We only fool ourselves by thinking we can find safety by isolating ourselves from others. Isolation is settling for a life in prison rather than a life of freedom, and a life in prison is a life of suffering. It is time to begin tearing down the bars of our self-made prison cells. It is time to overcome our denial.

Faith Traditions and the Meaning of Suffering

Because we have limited intelligence, we cannot fully understand the nature of the Higher Power. We speak different languages and we have many names for the Higher Power—Yahweh, God, Allah, Spirit, Father, Lord, and others. Many of us have turned to religion to help us understand why there is suffering in the world. Each of the great religious traditions confronts this problem in its own way.

The Christian, Islamic, and Jewish traditions each teach spiritual and emotional healing through prayer, meditation, and self-awareness. The followers of these faiths worship the same Higher Power but use different names—God, Allah, Yahweh. They are branches of the same tree, each tracing their roots to

Abraham of the Bible. These religions share a common understanding that each of us must submit to the will of the Higher Power. Christianity, Judaism, and Islam see this world as a battleground between good and evil, where evil is often cleverly disguised in our midst. Believers must be vigilant in prayer and meditation in order to distinguish "good" from "evil." Self-esteem is a good thing, but there is a fine line between self-esteem and inappropriate pride. An abundance of food is a good thing, but damaging our bodies through overeating is not. Sexual pleasure is a good thing, but its pursuit can also lead to much suffering. In our modern society, we are constantly bombarded with advertisements for new and improved products or services. In and of themselves, these are neither good nor bad, but they can easily become false gods, distracting us from the will of the Higher Power. For Christians, Jews, and Muslims, a religious life means subjugation of our will to the will of the Higher Power. It means building a conscious connection with the Higher Power. When Christians, Jews, or Muslims confront pain and suffering, they should do so with the understanding that there is a reason for everything, including illness and pain.

The Buddha is regarded as the Enlightened One or the great teacher of the Buddhist faith. He taught that true awareness brings inner peace. Suffering, according to the Buddhist faith, is caused by our preoccupation with worldly concerns. The more we think about the past, worry about the future, and try to control life around us—the more we suffer. For Buddhists, religious practice is based in meditation, leading to self-awareness and detachment from worldly concerns. Many Buddhists prefer to use the word nonattachment rather than detachment, because they do not see themselves as detached from life and spirit. For Buddhists, to be enlightened they must learn to overcome the illusion of independence and come to know our true selves as part of a greater Being, Spirit or Consciousness.

33

According to the Hindu religion, each of us enters this world with strengths and weaknesses. Each of us has our own path to follow. Each of us must confront the obstacles that life hands us—including pain and suffering. For Hindus, there are many paths and many religious practices. For some, meditation is the right way. For others, it may be a commitment to their work. By following religious teachings and practices, each of us grows spiritually. Hindus believe in reincarnation. They believe that we can be reincarnated into a higher level of consciousness, better able to deal with the next life if we are committed to self-awareness and self-improvement.

No matter what our religious beliefs, we need to move beyond the idea that all of our suffering is caused by a physical problem. Medical conditions cause pain, but much of our suffering is self-imposed. Since we believe in a Power greater than ourselves, we must accept the fact that our lives are part of a plan that is beyond our understanding. We need to develop a proper perspective about what is truly important in life— avoiding the traps of negative feelings such as fear, bitterness, and jealousy. In order to recover from our suffering, we must overcome our isolation and take our place in the world. As we do so, we begin to live in the present, fretting less about the past or worrying about the future. We have chosen to come together because we were meant to help one and other. We can overcome our fears, worries, and bitterness. We come together to ask the Higher Power's guidance so that we can find true meaning in our lives.

Fear

Most of us have at least heard of, if not seen, the *Star Wars* movies. However, most people are not aware that this outer space drama was written with a specific intent of increasing young people's spiritual awareness. In writing his screenplay,

George Lucas consulted with Joseph Campbell, a well-known authority on ancient myth and symbol. Lucas recognized that there are universal truths, and that myths can help us understand these truths. Star Wars is fiction, but it there is truth in its message. Like the old Greek myths, Lucas's heroes struggle to overcome great obstacles, often suffering in the process. Lucas names the Higher Power the Force. Though the *Star Wars* heroes do not understand the Force, they must attune themselves to its will. They set aside their own concerns, risking their lives to be true to the Light [good] Side of the Force. As the ancients learned from mythological stories about their gods, we can learn from Lucas's futuristic saga.

The *Star Wars* outer space drama begins when Jedi knights—warriors with special psychic and physical powers— are sent to escort Queen Amadala to an interplanetary council meeting where she intends to seek help in defending her planet against attack by an evil trade federation. Unfortunately, her spaceship becomes disabled. The queen and her Jedi knight escorts are forced to seek repairs on a remote planet ruled by gangsters and thugs. A young slave boy, Anakin Skywalker, and his mother befriend the Queen and the Jedi. After many adventures, the group escapes the planet taking Anakin with them. Sadly, they must leave behind Anakin's mother.

Young Anakin wants to become a Jedi. Before he can do so, a special council of Jedi knights must determine his fitness for training. Yoda, the most senior of the Jedi, senses that Anakin is fearful about the mother he left behind. Yoda says, "Afraid, to lose her, I think? Fear is the path to the Dark Side. Fear leads to anger... anger leads to hate... hate leads to suffering."

Indeed, fear becomes Anakin's undoing, and he gradually turns away from the Light side of the Force. Eventually he becomes the dreaded Darth Vader—part man, part machine, cloaked in black and dedicated to serving the powers of darkness. When Anakin Skywalker becomes Darth Vader, he loses his freedom. Though still a powerful warrior, Vader is forced to serve at the will of an evil emperor. Vader lives in a prison of his own making. He is isolated from family and friends. His skin is replaced by armor, his face with a mask. He has little feelings for others.

In the last episode of *Star Wars*, we learn that there remains a spark of goodness in Darth Vader. He chooses to sacrifice his own life for that of his son, Luke Skywalker. Because he is wearing an armored mask, Vader's vision is distorted. Vader asks his son to remove the mask, knowing that this will hastens his death, As he lies dying at his son's feet, Vader is able to see the goodness in his son's face. In the end, good triumphs over evil. Freedom triumphs over tyranny. Love triumphs over fear.

Those of us who saw the Star Wars movies easily identify with the young, talented Anakin Skywalker—full of energy and enthusiasm. Like Anakin, we too were young, energetic and enthusiastic. Like Anakin, we may have held fear in our hearts and allowed it to make us bitter. Like Anakin, we may have turned to the Dark Side when we cut ourselves off from sources of love and hope. Unlike Anakin, we do not have to wait for death to make amends. We do not have to become an isolated, tormented, suffering Darth Vader. We can choose the way of Luke Skywalker, and attune ourselves to the Light Side of the Force—our Higher Power.

Sorrow—Neither Depression nor Suffering

Just as physical pain is different from suffering, sorrow is also different from depression. Sorrow comes from feeling loss in our lives. We feel sorrow or grief when a loved one dies. We feel sorrow when we leave a job we enjoy. We feel sorrow when our children go off to college. We feel sorrow when we are no longer able to do the things we once could. Sorrow is natural. Sorrow is part of life. Sorrow is healthy because it makes us stronger and sorrow can help us learn to cope with the inevitable losses that are part of living. Hopefully, we learned healthy grieving from our parents. Our first experience with death and dying might have been when a relative died. It might also have been the grief of losing a family pet. We may have experienced many losses as children, and those early experiences were meant to teach us about loss and about its acceptance.

It is okay to feel sorrow over loss of bodily function caused by our medical conditions. It is okay to feel sorrow over the fact that pain limits our activities. Sorrow is not a disease that needs medication. In fact, treating it with medication can actually numb our feelings and interfere with the emotional growth that normally accompanies grieving.

Depression is not healthy, nor is it the same as sorrow or grief. Depression does not lead to emotional growth. Feelings of hopelessness and low self-worth that often accompany depression are not positive. Depression is a form of suffering that keeps us locked in the past and interferes with our recovery. When we are depressed, we withdraw from relationships and question our faith and our future. When we are depressed, we become self-absorbed. When we are depressed, we lose our conscious connection with the Higher Power. In order to move along in our recovery, we must learn to recognize the difference between healthy sorrow and unhealthy, negative reactions to our losses.

The Higher Power's Plan for Us

Some of us may be angry with the Higher Power because we were not protected when we were children. We may ask why a Higher Power would allow adults to take advantage of us. Why do bad things happen to good people? Why is there evil in the world? Since we are limited in our ability to understand the meaning of life, we often turn to parables, myths, and allegories to help answer these difficult questions.

The *Bible* begins with the story of Genesis—of how God created the universe. In the beginning, there was darkness—a symbol of ignorance and evil. God said, "Let there be light," and God saw it was good. Later, God decided to create "people in His own image." God created Adam and Eve, the first humans, and placed them in the Garden of Paradise. Even within the Garden, evil lurked in the form of the serpent-devil who tempted Adam and Eve into eating from the forbidden fruit.

There are many interpretations of the Genesis story. One interpretation is that Adam and Eve did not become fully human until they ate from the "tree of the knowledge of good and evil." Before they ate the fruit, they did not have to plow the fields, forage for food, or even carry water. All of their needs were met. Without needing to work at all, they were certainly not human in the same way that we are. But once they ate the forbidden fruit, they became self-conscious—that is, they became aware of themselves. For the first time, they saw themselves as they really were, and they were immediately ashamed of their nakedness.

Of all the animals in creation, it appears that only humans have the capacity for self-consciousness or self-awareness. We must work to survive. We must make choices about good and evil. Like Adam and Eve, we experience guilt and shame, happiness and suffering. Nothing in Genesis or other creation stories implies that the Higher Power has preordained everything that humans will experience. Our pain was not preordained. Pain is just a fact of creation, like birth, aging, and death.

Creation continues to unfold. The universe continues to expand. The battle between good and evil continues. This battle takes place in the lives of each one of us. As we become increasing self-aware, and more conscious of the Higher Power's will for us, we become better at recognizing right from wrong. As we grow in spirit, we begin to heal, our families begin to heal, and the world becomes a better place for all of humankind. Throughout history, men and women have freely chosen love and truth [good] over fear and falsehood [evil]. It is through the courageous acts of individuals, many of whom were afflicted with physical pain, that we come to understand truth. The Higher Power works within our lives, not apart.

There may be some among us who doubt that we continue to evolve in body, mind, and spirit. They may doubt that we have benefited from the struggles of our ancestors. We need to remember that many things we now consider wrong were once considered right—evils such as slavery, polygamy and domination of women by men. Time did not stand still when the *Bible* was written. If it did, we would still find these practices acceptable because they were practiced when the Bible was written and for many centuries afterwards. Each one of us has an important part to play in this evolution. We have a choice. We play the role of the hero in the drama of life— guided by the power of love, we can overcome the traps of negative thinking and negative behavior, or we can remain trapped in our isolation, fear, and resentments.

Serenity Prayer

God grant me the serenity to accept the things I cannot change; the courage to change the things I can; and the wisdom to know the difference.

Many Twelve Step meetings close with the Serenity Prayer. For those suffering with chronic pain, this prayer can have special meaning. We must learn to accept the things that we cannot change in our lives, including the fact that we have painful physical conditions. But there are many things we can change, and with the help of the Higher Power, we can overcome our negative attitudes, beliefs, and behaviors. Doing so will greatly reduce our suffering.

Inspirational Reading—Nelson Mandela

"There is no easy walk to freedom anywhere, and many of us will have to pass through the valley of the shadow of death again and again before we reach the mountaintop of our desires."

"The greatest glory in living lies not in never falling, but in rising every time we fall."

It is hard to image growing up in poverty, with no shoes to wear, and no modern conveniences. It is hard to imagine being considered a "third class" citizen—not allowed rights reserved for the ruling class. It is even harder to imagine the suffering of having to spend most of your adult life being beaten and ridiculed in prison. Living such a life, we could easily become consumed by anger, bitterness, and pain. What kind of individual, treated so badly, would find it in his heart to forgive his enemies as he walked out of prison? Mandela is such a man.

Mandela rose from utter poverty to become the first Black president of South Africa and a winner of the Nobel Peace Prize. He worked as a herd boy, and he did not own a pair of shoes until he was sixteen years old. Because their family was so poor, Nelson Mandela's mother decided to move to a Methodist mission where the family would be provided food and shelter. The missionaries recognized young Mandela's talents and, at their urging, he attended a one-room Western-style school. Mandela later attended college and law school.

In an effort to fight segregation, Nelson Mandela embarked on a nonviolent campaign against the South African apartheid system. He traveled around the country, recruiting volunteers to break immoral apartheid laws through civil disobedience such as passing through "Whites only" entrances to railroad stations and defying curfews. During one of these nonviolent actions, Mandela was arrested—the first of many arrests and indignities he would endure. In 1962, he chose to defend himself at his trial. During this defense he said, "During my lifetime I have dedicated myself to this struggle of the African people. I have fought against White domination, and I have fought against Black domination. I have cherished the ideal of a democratic and free society in which all persons live together in harmony and with equal opportunities. It is an ideal, which I hope to live for and to achieve. But if needs be, it is an ideal for which I am prepared to die."

While in prison, Mandela came to embody the struggle of all oppressed African peoples. When he was finally released in 1990, he resumed the work he had begun almost four decades earlier. In 1994, Nelson Mandela became the first democratically elected President of South Africa. Rather than persecuting those who had imprisoned and tortured him, he chose a path of forgiveness. He instituted a Truth and

41

Reconciliation Commission that gave all those who committed crimes, both White and Black South Africans, a chance to come forward and admit their wrongdoings as part of the national healing process. Nelson Mandela overcame fear, anger, pain, and humiliation. Along the way, he brought peace to himself and to his nation.

Prayer for the Third Step

I have tried to control the uncontrollable for too long. Help me remove the blinders of self-will. Help me see what is true. Free me from self-pity, from resentment, from discontent. Allow me to see what you would have me do and grant me the strength to follow through.

Exercises for the Third Step

Religious Practice

Religion can be a source of great strength for those who have strong faith beliefs. If you believe in the teachings of a particular religion, set aside time each day to pray for a better understanding of the Higher Power's will for you. Make an effort to regularly attend your church, synagogue, temple or mosque. In order to gain a deeper understanding of your faith, join discussion or study groups. Seek out members of your faith community that have had to deal with adversity and learn how they managed.

Mindful Meditation

When most people think of meditation, they think of transcendental or similar meditation techniques involving repeating of a phrase or mantra. In mindful meditation, there is no mantra and no special breathing technique other than relaxed, slow, deep breathing. All forms of meditation help relax muscles, and muscle relaxation often decreases pain, but mindfulness is one of the best researched of all methods. Mindfulness brings awareness to the present moment. It helps us learn to live in the "here and now." It helps us become less impulsive and reactive by learning that feelings and thoughts do not require immediate action. With practice, we find ourselves able to remain calm, despite the whirlwind of activity around us. No longer blown to and fro by what others say and do, intrusive memories of our past, or worries about the future, we are able to follow a straighter course. No longer distracted by the noise around us, we can take the time to listen to the voice of the Higher Power guiding us on our journey.

Before beginning mindful meditation, it is important to assume a comfortable position. There are many online resources that describe mindful meditation, and most suggest meditation sitting in a chair. Because some of us have back pain, it may serve us better to use an alternative posture—the constructive resting position. This position has a number of benefits including relaxing spinal muscles and releasing tension in the psoas muscle—common contributing factors in back pain. Rest your head on a small pillow, folded towel, or stack of books about two inches high—raising your head just enough to keep your neck from arching back. Rest only the back of your head on the pillow; your neck should not make contact with the pillow. The ideal height varies from person to person. If your head is tipping forward (chin to throat) it is too high. If your head is tilting back (chin higher than forehead) then it is too low. Draw your knees up to the ceiling, such that your feet are resting flat on the floor. Space your heels approximately 12-16 inches away from your buttocks. Your feet should be wide enough apart so your legs do not flop apart, if anything, they may be tipped a little to the midline. Do not push your low back to the floor, rather just rest in the position.

Close your eyes, but in a relaxed manner. Your eyelids should be barely touching. Take full, but normal, breaths. Become aware of your breathing. Become aware of the fresh oxygen-rich air filling your lungs and the stale, carbon dioxide-laden air leaving your lungs. As you breathe in and out, you should become increasingly aware of your thoughts and feelings. You do not want to judge your thoughts or feelings in any way. You want merely to name them when they enter your consciousness and then let them go.

When a thought or feeling enters your mind, you should give it a name and repeat this name in your mind. You then return to concentrating on your breathing until another thought or feeling enters your consciousness. It will be difficult at first, since thoughts and feeling will keep popping into your consciousness every few seconds. With time, you will relax and your racing thoughts will slow down.

Example: While you are breathing, you hear a bird chirping. You say to yourself, "bird." You resume your breathing. You then become aware of a pain in your back, and say to yourself, "back." Do not say "pain"; rather simply note the location of your pain. You resume breathing and begin thinking about your job. Say to yourself, "job", and so on. Let the thoughts come and go without judgment. You will begin to notice that the thoughts come further and further apart.

As you repeat this exercise daily, you will learn detachment from your thoughts, pain, and negative feelings. You will also become more aware of those things that clutter your mind and learn better ways of confronting life's challenges.

Progressive Muscle Relaxation

Progressive muscle relaxation is another exercise that helps to reduce pain. It involves progressively contracting and then relaxing specific muscle groups, usually beginning with the forehead and working down to the toes. There are many variations of this and other relaxation techniques. It is beyond the scope of this book to provide detailed instruction on mind-body exercises. However, every library has books that describe progressive relaxation as well as meditation, yoga, and other techniques to improve health. Also, information is readily available online. If one technique does not seem to work for you, try another.

Chapter 4

Becoming Who We Really Are

Chronic Pain Step 4: Made a searching and fearless morale inventor of ourselves.

Melissa's Story

"I am only in my thirties, but I was told I had the cervical spine of a sixty-year-old. I had tried all kinds of treatments, but I was still in pain. I needed more and more pain medication, and my life was getting out of control.

My mother had been an alcoholic. When I was a girl, I had to help take care of my little brother. A few months before I first went to see the doctor for neck pain, my brother committed suicide. He was a drug addict, and had just recently gotten clean. I was devastated. It was like part of my heart was ripped out of me.

The doctor told me that I would always have neck pain because of arthritis, but that I could find ways to decrease the pain. The doctor said that my worry and stress added to my pain, so he referred me to a pain psychologist who taught me relaxation techniques. In therapy I learned that I magnified problems. My therapist asked me to make an honest assessment of both my strengths and weaknesses At first, I could think of little that was positive in my life. I believed I was a poor wife, an inadequate mother, and that I had failed my brother.

Many months have passed since then. I no longer need pain medications. I have learned a great deal about myself, including the fact that I have many strengths: survival skills, intelligence, strong work ethic, compassion, and a desire to help others. I also have weakness: worry, perfectionism, and excessive caretaking. Understanding who I am has allowed me to change how I cope with chronic pain. It has also helped me learn to deal with other challenges I face in my life. I have grown in so many ways. Sometimes, I think that my neck pain was a blessing in disguise."

Life—A Journey of Discovery

Life is a journey. We entered into life as newborns completely dependent on others, hardly aware of more than our bodily sensations and immediate surroundings. When we were toddlers, each day brought new surprises. We were amazed and delighted at our new discoveries. As school age children, we had less time for play. Many of us enjoyed learning. For some, school was an unwelcome obligation that deprived us of playtime. Along the way, many of us lost the joy of learning and discovery that we once had as children.

Somewhere between childhood and adulthood, we began to ask ourselves difficult questions about the meaning of life. How do I fit in? Why is there suffering in the world? Some of us sought answers to these questions in books, college courses, or religious practice, but the answers we found were never complete. The truth is that each of us must find our own answers to these questions because each of us views the world from a unique perspective. No two individuals, not even identical twins, share the exact same perspective. Each of us brings to our experience our own personal history. Each reacts to the world around us differently. Our beliefs and our feelings greatly influence how we see the world.

We have all heard that optimistic people see the world through rose-colored glasses. They see more good than bad in their lives. Few of us with chronic pain are inclined toward optimism. But we need a more positive attitude in order to proceed with our recovery. To get a better understanding of reality, we need to understand how our beliefs and feelings color our view of the world. In order to do this, we need to become more self-aware. And as we become more aware, we will learn that we can change our beliefs and change how we react to our feelings. With time, we can begin to see the world in a different, more positive light.

Getting in Touch with our Feelings

As infants, we made no attempt to control our emotions. If we were hungry, we cried. If we were tired, we were grumpy. If we were happy, we smiled. Along the way, children learn to hide some of their feelings and emotions from others. This is a natural part of social development. As an example, at some point our parents told us to "stop crying" or "stop complaining" when we were hurting. Rather than face our parents' reproaches, we learned to do just that, but we still had our feelings. With time, we learned to keep feelings to ourselves. For some of us, trapped—or so-called repressed feelings became a major problem. To better understand how repressed feelings affect our pain, compare the two examples below:

Example 1: Dick enters the house at the end of a long, tiring day at work. He mumbles a "hello" to his wife as he takes a beer from the refrigerator, sits on the sofa, and clicks on the TV.

Jane: "Did you have a bad day, honey?"

Dick: "Who said I had a bad day?"

Jane: "You seem angry, honey."

Dick slams his beer down on the coffee table.

Dick: "I never said I was angry! I'm fine!"

Example 2: Dan enters the house at the end of a long workday. He mumbles a "hello" to his wife as he goes to refrigerator, takes out a beer, sits on the sofa, and clicks on the TV.

Gina: "Did you have a bad day, honey?"

Dan: "A bad day at this job? No, never. Being blamed for problems I didn't do is just loads of fun!"

Gina: "It's just a job. I appreciate what you do!"

Dan: "Thanks, sweetie."

Dan sits back in the couch and clicks on the TV.

In these two examples, Dick and Dan each had a bad day at work. In the first example, Dick repressed his anger and frustration, keeping it bottled-up inside of him all day. He might not have realized he was angry. When confronted by his wife, Dick denied that he was angry and vented at her. In the second example, Dan knew he had a tough day. He was able to keep his cool. He admitted to Gina that he was angry, and felt relieved to express his feelings. Like Dick and Dan, we have bad days at work and find ourselves stressed. We need to recognize what is really going on. We need to identify the specific emotions we are experiencing—negative emotions such as anger, sadness, guilt, fear, shame, or positive emotions such as joy and excitement. As we do so, we will learn that we do not have to immediately react to our feelings. Rather, we can choose among different ways to deal with them.

Each of us has a bit of Dick and Dan in us; it is only a matter of degree. Those of us with chronic pain are more likely to repress negative feelings such as anger and fear than others might. Those who were abused as children had little choice but to "deal with it" and did not learn healthy ways of expressing hurt, anger, or fear. Some of us were raised in households where parents did not openly express feelings, so we had difficulty learning healthy emotional expression. Now we must learn to share the facts of our lives, including our negative feelings with others.

As we progress in this program, we want to become more like Dan. We want to recognize our feelings and express them openly and honestly. Dan may not have been comfortable expressing his frustrations to his work supervisor, but he trusted Gina and shared his feelings with her. For many of us, trust is difficult. Some of us have a habit of trusting people, and we are hurt often when our trust was broken. Some of us trust no one, so we never share our feelings. Not only must we learn to recognize our feelings, we must learn whom we can trust. Twelve Step meetings help us learn to trust. In Twelve Step meetings, we remain anonymous and no one is permitted to comment on what another has said. Everyone has an equal opportunity to share feelings, and everyone's feelings are validated when the group says, "Thanks for sharing." We learn to listen attentively to those who have made the most progress in their own recovery. We learn that these are individuals whom we can trust, and we may ask one of them to serve as our sponsor—someone who can guide us on our journey.

Learning That Feelings Belong to Us

Our feelings are within us. They do not exist in the outside world. We can react to our feelings in different ways, or choose not to react at all. When we have physical pain, we can react in different ways, as demonstrated in this example:

Example: Dick walked into his kitchen after a tough day at work. He went to get a beer from the refrigerator, but he does not notice the spilled juice on the kitchen floor. He slips and falls on his behind, cursing angrily "God D_ _ _ n it!" Slapping his palm against the floor he adds, "Who the hell spilled juice on the floor?"

Of course, yelling and hitting the floor did little to change the fact that Dick bruised his tail bone. His pain is real, but he could have chosen to deal with this pain in a number of ways. He did not have to slap the floor in anger. This only made his hand hurt! He could have gotten up and "walked it off" as football players do, or applied ice, or taken an aspirin. Instead, he screamed and then interrogated family members to find out who spilled the juice. Since no one would admit to it, Dick remained angry and continued to sulk. For the next couple of days, he would think about the incident each time he opened the refrigerator or when he had to reposition himself to take weight off his sore tail bone. His anger became resentment. He thought to himself, "I don't get any respect in this family." Dick's anger, resentment, and blame did nothing to help with his sore behind; in fact, his negative feelings just added to suffering.

From time to time, we all act the way Dick did. While it is true that the direct cause of Dick's pain was his fall, neither the kitchen floor nor the person who spilled the juice made him angry. When we say that other people make us feel sad, angry, resentful, or nervous, we delude ourselves. No one makes us feel our emotions. We can learn to change how we react to other people's actions. In our example, Dick was wasting time and energy stewing about who spilled the juice. Without realizing it, he was letting another person in his family control his thoughts and feelings.

Just as Dick's pain and anger belong to him, our feelings belong to us. Each time we assume someone makes us feel a certain way, we lose power to that person because we let him or her control our lives. When we believe that others cause us to feel and act the way we do, we limit our own freedom. Since none of us really wants to be controlled by others, we try to avoid emotional suffering by changing the world around us. We try to change our family, friends, bosses, coworkers, and anybody else we think is causing our suffering. We mistakenly believe that if we can change them, we can make our negative feelings go away. This strategy is doomed to failure because our negative feelings are in us—not in them. We cannot begin to see reality, until we recognize feelings for what they are— just feelings. We do not need to change others—we need to change ourselves!

Anger

Anger is a natural and appropriate human emotion, but many of us never learned to deal with anger in healthy ways. We may have grown up in a household where a parent had explosive rage, so we became afraid of anger. We might have had parents that did not allow us to express our anger; children who are not allowed to express anger sometimes feel guilty when they are angry, since they learn that anger was bad. If we were not allowed to express anger towards our parents, we may have learned to misdirect our anger towards others. Some of us are so afraid of anger that we do not even realize when we are angry. Instead, anger turns into simmering resentment that occasionally boils over into rage. We need to understand the ways anger might be affecting our lives. Repressed anger keeps us from becoming honest with ourselves and with others.

The word "soma" means "body" in Greek. Psychologists use the term "somatization" to describe the process of emotional conflict or stress causing bodily symptoms. Repressed anger exacerbates any bodily pain, and often causes headaches, irritable bowel syndrome, sexual difficulties, rashes, sleep problems, and a host of other medical problems. In order to recover from repressed anger, we must first learn to accept that we are angry. It is okay to be angry. The problem is not anger, but how we express anger. Repressed anger not only causes physical harm, but it also harms our relationships with other people. If we learn to deal effectively with anger, we can use it as a force for change in our lives and in society. When we repress or keep feelings locked inside of us, we experience more pain.

Just as suffering is not a natural consequence of pain, resentment is not a natural consequence of anger. If we are angry with someone, we must first accept the fact that we are angry. If we feel that someone has hurt us in some way, we need to ask ourselves if it is appropriate to let that person know how we feel. Even in work situations, letting your supervisors know you are angry is usually okay.

Example: Jane's supervisor yells at her because she made a mistake. Yelling back at her supervisor is not okay, since this will only make matters worse (and she might lose her job). Keeping her anger hidden from her boss may lead to resentment, work dissatisfaction, and increased physical pain. If her supervisor is a reasonable person, Jane might say, "I know I made a mistake, and I will try to do better next time. When you yelled at me, my feelings were hurt. If I make a mistake again, I would appreciate it if you would pull me aside right away and let me know." If Jane approached her supervisor in this way, she might get a response such as, "I am sorry I yelled. I was having a bad day."

There is little to lose in sharing our feelings with another person, so long as we do so without accusation or threat. In the example above, Jane did not blame her supervisor for causing her hurt feelings. She accepted responsibility for making a mistake, and acknowledged her own feelings. Honest expression of feelings often improves our relationships with others. Healthy expression of anger releases us from tension, reduces our fear, and avoids resentment—a major cause of our suffering.

It is best to deal with angry feelings as directly and as soon as possible, although this is not always possible. Sometimes, our supervisors are not reasonable. Sometimes, we have little or no contact with the object of our anger. We might even be angry with a parent who is no longer living. In such cases, it is best to share our feelings with someone we trust. In doing so, we must be careful not to accuse the other person of causing our feelings. Rather, we should simply state what happened and how we feel. We must be careful not to blame. In this way, we learn that our feelings belong to us. Healthy sharing is one way to deal with our emotions.

Anger Exercise

Some of us sustained physical injuries at work or in a motor vehicle accident. Some of us were injured by the deliberate actions of another person. We may have suffered emotionally and financially because of our injuries. We may have seen doctors for pain management, only to have our pain increase during treatment. We may feel that our family and friends abandoned us after we were injured. We have many reasons to be angry. The problem is not with anger, but with keeping our anger locked inside, as this only increases our suffering. In this exercise, we identify our resentments.

For each category below, list as many examples as possible of how you hold onto resentments. Be as specific as possible (if you are angry with a person at work, write down the name of the person, not "work").

Friends

Family

Current Employer

Past Employer

Healthcare (e.g. doctors)

Religious Institutions

Government

Other

Shame

Guilt is a healthy response to doing something wrong. If we use our painful medical condition as an excuse to act badly, we should feel guilty. Some of us use pain as an excuse for not spending time with our families. We might use our medical condition as a way to get attention. We might be angry with a member of our family and use pain as an excuse for avoiding them. We might sometimes wallow in self-pity. We might feel guilty about ignoring family obligations, isolating ourselves from our families, or staying stuck in self-pity. Guilt is about taking responsibility for things we have done. When we feel guilty, we are getting the message that we did something wrong and now must make amends.

Shame is entirely different. When we feel shame, we feel that we are the problem, not our bad behavior. Some of us were shamed in childhood and never learned the difference between healthy guilt and shame. Because we might not know better, we could be shaming our own children without even realizing it. The following example helps explain the difference between guilt and shame.

Example: While walking on the sidewalk with her mother, three-year-old Penelope steps off the curb and into the street. Penelope's mother uses this incident as an opportunity to teach Penelope that it is not safe to walk in the street. There are many ways of dealing with this situation. Two are described below:

One way might be for her mother to say, "Penelope, never walk into the street again: that is a very, very bad thing you did. It is dangerous. You could be hit by a car."

Another way might be to spank Jane and say, "You are a very, very bad girl, Penelope, never walk into the street again. You could be hit by a car."

Teaching right and wrong is a parental responsibility. It may seem like the only difference between these two approaches is that in one example Penelope was spanked, but not in the other, but there is another important difference. In the first example, Penelope's mother tells her that she did a bad thing—stepping into the street. In the other example, she tells Penelope that she is a bad girl because she stepped into the street. One way teaches healthy guilt—if Penelope continues to walk into the street or do other bad things, she will feel remorse for doing wrong, and she will face repercussions. The other way teaches shame—if Penelope's mother continues to call her a "bad girl," Penelope will come to believe that she is a bad girl, and that she is the problem. Shame leaves her feeling put down. If she believes she is bad, she will also believe she is undeserving of love. Without a healthy sense of guilt, some children come to believe that doing bad things is expected of them. Children taught to feel shame instead of healthy guilt are at higher risk for low self-esteem, drug abuse, dependent relationships, and conduct problems.

In recent years, millions of people have become fascinated with reality TV shows. One popular show's premise is that contestants are organized into tribes living on an island. Tribal members cast lots to decide who should or who should not stay on an island. The TV producers carefully pick individuals whose feelings are not likely to be hurt when banished. With each weekly episode, devoted followers of the series speculated as to who will be voted off the island. .

In many cultures, banishment or shunning is used as the ultimate form of punishment. It can be so powerful that those shunned by society have been known to die because they believed they could not live without the support of the group. In passing this sentence on someone, the group would have judged the individual as so bad or dangerous that the group had no choice but banishment.

Psychologists who observe animal behavior tell us that shame plays an important role in keeping social order within animal groups. Those of us who own dogs easily recognize shame in our canine companions. When scolded, dogs cower—lowering their heads, retreating, and putting their tails between their legs. This is submissive behavior. Since dogs in the wild live in packs, they must be submissive to the top dog. Shame keeps the dogs in line by maintaining order in the pack. When we use shame to keep order in our homes or our society, we are following our animal or lower instincts, versus our human or higher instincts. As sons and daughters of a Higher Power, we are all created equal. We do not need to shame one another in order to establish order in our society. When societies put down a particular group, they rule by fear, not love. As an example, the Nazi movement was based upon the false belief in superior and inferior racial groups. Nazis used this false belief as the reason to shame and, ultimately, to kill those who did not agree with them.

Shame is the root of much evil in our world, and also the root of much of our own suffering. Just because someone puts us down, that does not mean that we are inferior in any way. Shame is a horrible feeling. When we are ashamed, we feel that there is something fundamentally wrong with us. All humans do bad things, yet many of us are unable to forgive ourselves for even the simplest of mistakes. Since we cannot forgive ourselves, we continually think about the mistakes we made. This keeps us stuck in the past, making it difficult for us to move forward with our lives.

Avoiding Conflict

Some people handle conflict better than others do. Sometimes, conflict escalates into confrontation. For many of us, even little conflicts may knock us off balance. We continue to fret over our problems. We listen to the voices inside our heads that criticize us for making mistakes or criticize others for their actions.

While the saying, "Sticks and stones can break my bones, but words can never hurt me," may be true for some, it certainly does not apply to those of us who are shame-ridden. The fact is that cruel words hurt so much because part of us actually believes that they are true. While it may have been our parents who initially told us we were bad little boys and girls, our shame can be triggered by any conflict. When we obsess over incidents, we are doing the job of shaming once done by our parents or other authority figures. Naturally, those of us overwrought with shame are more apt to have problems when in conflict with authority figures, as in the example that follows:

Penelope hears the siren of police car; looking in her mirror, she sees flashing lights right behind her and glances at her speedometer. She is doing 35-mph in a 15-mph zone. She is almost paralyzed by the feeling that she has been caught doing something terribly wrong. She pulls over and takes out her license and registration. The officer asks, "How fast do you think you were going?" Penelope's mouth is dry, but she answers, "I am not sure, officer." The officer replies, "You were going 35 in a 15 zone. You should know better: this is a school zone. You could have injured a child. I will have to give you a ticket." Penelope nods, lowering her head in submission to authority.

Someone with healthy guilt would accept responsibility for speeding and be more careful in the future. After all, this is not the end of the world. Many drivers exceed the speed limit from time to time, and a few receive tickets as a result. Penelope did not intentionally speed in the school zone; she just didn't see the sign. In the example above, Penelope is less likely to let it go than others because she is stuck in shame. Over the next few days, she may think about the incident, having little control over when it enters into his thoughts. Unconsciously, she feels that she was caught doing something shameful—just as little Penelope might have felt when she was shamed for stepping off the curb into the street! To avoid the feeling of shame she might make excuses, such as the fact that the speed limit was not clearly marked, or that she was in a hurry because she was late for an appointment, or that she was worried about something important. She might blame the police officer for not giving her a break. It is difficult for anyone with shame to accept imperfection. Penelope may continue to stew about the ticket for a few more weeks. If Penelope has back pain, all of this stress will make her back feel worse. Of course, none of Penelope's obsession with this incident does any good at all. It does not change the fact that she got a ticket. Shame keeps Penelope from acknowledging that she did something wrong. It keeps her stuck in the past and causes suffering.

Fear of Criticism

A recent survey asked people what social situation they most feared. At the top of the list was the fear of public speaking. Why are so many people afraid of speaking in front of groups? One reason is fear of criticism. This is the same reason why so many people do not want to participate in Twelve Step recovery groups. Participation requires public speaking, but overcoming fear is essential to recovery.

We know that we need to share our thoughts and feelings with others. Recovery groups are safe places to share. Because Twelve Step programs are anonymous, last names are never used. At each meeting, those present are reminded to not repeat what was said at a meeting. No one attending a meeting should have to fear that others could violate their trust. Since Twelve Step meetings do not allow cross-talk, no one is allowed to comment or criticize what another person says. After someone speaks, no matter what he or she may have said, the group responds with the affirmation, "Thank you for sharing." In this way, everyone in the group is treated with respect. Meetings usually close with the statement, "Take what you want and leave the rest." This statement reinforces the understanding that it is okay to judge what we hear at

STEPHEN COLAMECO, MD, M.ED.

meetings, but not okay to judge who said them. By speaking at meetings, we overcome the fear and shame that cause so much of our suffering.

Isolation

Chronic pain can lead to isolation. We may be irritable and not want others' company. We may be ashamed of our illness or disability. When we isolate, we cut ourselves off from the sources of love and support that we require in order to heal. Studies have shown that pain gets better when we spend more time in activities we enjoy, especially if we are doing them with people we love. In order to recover from emotional suffering, we need to increase our contact with others. At first, this may seem difficult. If we feel guilty because we have ignored relationships, it is best to be honest and direct with those we neglected. As an example, we might say, "I am sorry I have not spent much time with you lately. I have not been feeling well and wanted to be alone. Now I am feeling better, and I am beginning to realize that I need your friendship." We must make a commitment to spend more time with friends and family. Recovery helps us overcome our isolation and open ourselves to the love that surrounds us.

Inflicting Pain on Ourselves

Although we do not fully understand the connection between chronic pain and stress, we do know that many chronic pain sufferers were victims of physical or emotional abuse. Some studies have found that over half of chronic pain sufferers were abused—especially women. Chronic pain patients are also more likely to have major depression and problems with drinking or drugs. Stress is a major contributor to chronic pain.

As difficult as it may be to understand, individuals with serious psychiatric problems sometimes find relief from their intense negative feelings by hurting themselves. Their shame can be so toxic that they cut or burn themselves. They may hear voices that tell them to hurt themselves. These are very disturbed individuals who require intensive psychiatric care, but we can learn a lot about abnormal psychology by studying such extreme cases of self-abuse.

Many victims of child abuse find themselves in abusive adult relationships. It may seem peculiar that someone who was abused as a child would tolerate the same kind of behavior as an adult. However, victims of abuse may believe that a bad relationship is better than no relationship at all. They may feel undeserving of a loving relationship, or be too afraid to risk real intimacy. Abuse victims need emotional healing in order to overcome pain and suffering.

While few of us have ever cut or burned ourselves, we often criticize ourselves because we have limitations or make simple mistakes. Beating up on ourselves is yet another form of self-abuse. As we move forward in the twelve steps, we will learn to distinguish healthy guilt from unhealthy shame. Psychotherapy is the primary treatment for overcoming shame, but medications can also be helpful. Medications may be necessary for some people to successfully work the twelve steps. Certain types of antidepressants reduce shame, or at least reduce the impact of shame-triggered self-criticism. Those who benefit from these medications notice that while they still have negative thoughts, the thoughts do not spiral out of control. They are able to dismiss their negative thoughts without beating up on themselves.

In recent years, antidepressant mediations have received approval from the U.S. Food and Drug Administration for the treatment of chronic pain. The exact mechanisms for the antidepressant and pain alleviating actions of these medications are unknown. Some experts believe these medications work by relieving the depression and anxiety experienced by patients in pain. Others proposed pain relieving properties result from activating brain pathways to directly dampen pain signals in the central nervous system. Unlike opioids, tranquilizers and some muscle relaxants, antidepressant medications are not addicting and may help alleviate physical and emotional pain.

Inspirational Reading—Mahatma Gandhi

"The weak can never forgive. Forgiveness is the attribute of the strong."

"An eye for an eye makes the whole world blind."

"Fear is not a disease of the body; fear kills the soul."

"Whenever I see an erring man, I say to myself I have also erred; when I see a lustful man I say to myself, so was I once; and in this way I feel kinship with everyone in the world and feel that I cannot be happy without the humblest of us being happy."

"Suffering has its well-defined limits. Suffering can be both wise and unwise, and when the limit is reached, to prolong it would be not unwise, but the height of folly."

"You can chain me, you can torture me, you can even destroy this body, but you will never imprison my mind."

Mahatma Gandhi knew about physical and emotional suffering. He was born 1869, when India was still a British colony. He was a shy boy and an average student. As was the Hindu custom, he entered into an arranged marriage when he was only 13. In 1887, he went to England to study law and, after completing his studies returned to India to practice law. The young Gandhi was very insecure. During his first jury trial, he became so nervous that he could not speak in the courtroom; another attorney had to finish the case for him. In 1893, he accepted a job in South Africa as a legal consultant, a position that did not require public speaking.

On arriving in South Africa, Gandhi faced discrimination because he was Indian and had a dark complexion. He had to travel in third class train compartments, was not allowed to walk on public footpaths, and had to abide by a curfew. It was in South Africa that Gandhi found his voice.

Gandhi discovered that when he was speaking from his heart, his voice never failed. His purpose in life was not to become a successful Indian lawyer. Gandhi's purpose was to speak on behalf of those who were oppressed by unjust laws. While in South Africa, he began to organize Indians against the discrimination laws of South Africa. Over the next decade, he became increasingly active in support of all human rights. During his stay in South Africa, Gandhi opened a hospital and founded an Indian language newspaper.

As a direct result of his nonviolent protest activities, Gandhi was often imprisoned. In order to strengthen his resolve, he chose to live a very simple life. He also decided to strengthen his spirit through self-discipline. He meditated, fasted often, and wore the rough, homespun clothes of India's lowest class—the untouchables. As Gandhi gained control over his emotions, he developed a clearer vision of how he was to proceed with his program of nonviolent confrontation through civil disobedience of unjust laws.

In 1914, Gandhi returned to India and founded an ashram, or religious community. Gandhi offered help to those in need, including the untouchables. In 1919, he organized a countrywide strike against British Imperial rule, a day during which workers prayed and fasted. This was one of many political actions undertaken by Gandhi. In 1922, he was sentenced to six years in prison, but was released in 1924 due to his poor health. Gandhi continued his civil disobedience campaigns against British rules. He was arrested twice more and fasted for long periods. His fasts were particularly effective because the British feared that a general uprising would occur should he die during a fast. Through Gandhi's efforts, Britain finally granted India its independence, and Gandhi was honored as father of the new nation. Gandhi is widely recognized as one of the greatest men of the twentieth century. He inspired civil rights leaders, such as Rev. Martin Luther King, to adopt nonviolent tactics. Gandhi turned shyness, insecurity, persecution, discomfort and pain into the strength that he needed to liberate his nation.

Prayer for the Fourth Step

I have added to my suffering through negative thoughts and behaviors. These mistakes were mine. I will begin a searching and fearless inventory of my strengths and weaknesses. I will write down my wrongs, but I will also include my good deeds. I pray for the strength to complete the task.

Exercise for the Fourth Step

All Twelve Step programs require a moral inventory. As an example, an alcoholic working the twelve steps of AA must list all of the things that he has done wrong or responsibilities he has neglected because of his drinking. In the Twelve Step approach to chronic pain, we make a list our ineffective coping behaviors rather than moral weaknesses as is customary in Twelve Step programs. We do this to identify those things about us that we need to change in order to overcome our suffering. All of us have coping strategies. Psychiatrists sometimes refer to them as defense mechanisms. We developed these coping strategies during our childhood, but they may not be serving us well as adults.

As an example, Jane was the daughter of an overly demanding mother. As a child, she became a perfectionist in order to please her mother. This unconscious strategy worked well in dealing with her mother's constant demands, but it became a liability in adulthood. As an adult, Jane is now married and works as a supervisor. She constantly worries about work deadlines and is too demanding of her subordinates. As a wife, she is irritated by her husband's habit of not completing projects. She spends a great deal of time trying to change her coworkers and her husband—to little effect, except for increasing her own stress. Perfectionism worked well in dealing with her mother, but not in dealing with her husband and coworkers.

Some of our coping behaviors are still useful, but others have become dysfunctional. Coping behaviors common to those with chronic pain are listed below. Honestly answer whether these coping behaviors apply to you. If they do apply, list ways in which they are no longer useful. Recognize that some of these same coping behaviors may also be strengths. We cannot just toss them away. We must learn to make gradual changes in our behavior, thus turning our weaknesses into strengths.

Control:

Negative aspects—Trying to control everything around us is a waste of time and energy. Have you wasted energy trying to control other people?

Positive aspects—Because some of us have become so skillful at manipulating situations, we have learned the art of influence. Influence is similar to control, but is not the same. Political lobbyists and salespeople must be skilled in the art of influence if they are to succeed. When we attempt to influence others, we are not upset when they do not act in the way we want; it is their choice, not ours. Have you developed the ability to influence others in positive ways?

Perfectionism:

Negative aspects—Since none of us is perfect, perfectionism dooms us to failure, convincing us of our low self-worth. Are you a perfectionist? Provide examples.

Positive aspects—Those of us who have striven to become perfect tend to be very conscientious in our duties. We often pay greater attention to detail than do others. These are traits that employers value. Are you a conscientious parent, partner, or worker?

Caretaking:

Negative aspects—Some of us are so attentive to the needs of others that we do not even recognize our own needs. Caretaking can keep us stuck in unhealthy relationships. If our needs are not met, we may become resentful, and this increases our suffering. Do you feel that you must take care of others in order to feel good about yourself? Provide examples where you neglected your own needs in a relationship.

Positive aspects—Some of us chose the helping professions because of our caretaking tendencies. Because we have suffered, we empathize with those who are suffering. There is nothing wrong with empathy or legitimate caretaking, as long as we do not lose track of our needs. Are there times when you provide care to others out of a need for approval versus out of genuine concern? Provide examples of legitimate caretaking.

People-pleasing:

Negative aspects—Some of us try desperately to be praised and to avoid criticism; we are "people pleasers." Like caretaking, people-pleasing keeps us from recognizing our own needs, and it gives our personal power over to those we must please. Do you sometimes act against your better judgment because you want to be liked or appreciated? Provide examples of people-pleasing.

Positive aspects—Most companies want their employees to exceed the expectations of their customers? Those of us who grew up as people-pleasers are very sensitive to customer needs. Are there times when you are courteous and sensitive to others' needs without compromising your own values?

Criticism:

Negative aspects—Some of us are overly critical of others and may be quick to find fault. Criticism of others keeps us from getting close to others. It allows us to avoid the risks associated with intimacy. It keeps people from knowing us and keeps us from knowing them. Are you overly critical of others? Give examples of how your criticism has affected your relationships.

Positive aspects—Critical thinking is essential to many jobs. Critical thinking can be channeled away from criticism of others, and into our professions. Scientists have highly developed critical thinking abilities. Do you have the ability to constructively criticize ideas or plans, without criticizing people? Provide examples.

Worry:

Negative aspects—Worry accomplishes very little. It gives us a false feeling of control. It adds to our stress and our pain. Are you a "worrier"? What do you worry about?

Positive aspects—Some worry is legitimate concern. We all would like our doctors to be concerned enough about us that they occasionally worry about our situation at times other than during office visits. Are you able to stop worrying enough to take a specific action? As an example, if you worry that your son is out too late, rather than fret, can you stop worrying by telling yourself you can call him in 30 minutes if he has not yet returned? Provide examples of legitimate concerns about others.

Chapter 5

Honesty—the First Step Towards Intimacy

Chronic Pain Step 5: Admitted to our Higher Power, to ourselves, and to another human being the exact nature of our wrong.

Paul's Story

"I am married and have a wonderful family. I had everything going my way, or so I thought. I was a police officer who loved his job—until I was injured my neck in a car accident. I ended up seeing orthopedic, neurosurgery and pain specialists. Along the way, I was prescribed a narcotic—oxycodone. Over time, I noticed I needed more and more of this pain medication to get the same effect. One day, I realized that I was addicted. I don't mean that I would get sick if I stopped the medicine; I mean I was taking more than I knew I should. The medication made me feel good. I was ashamed that this had happened to me. Can you imagine, going from a police officer who arrests drug addicts to becoming one? I was angry over what had happened to my life.

I entered a rehabilitation program that treated both chronic pain and addiction. The program included detoxification, physical therapy, counseling, acupuncture and meditation. In group sessions, we spent a lot of time talking about anger and resentment.

Two years later, I still have pain in my neck and need to take medication but not narcotics. I have learned to cope well with chronic pain and no longer see myself as a victim.

Giving up the Sick Role

Any time we try to change the way we live, we face conflict and stress because we have become accustomed to living a certain way. As an example, most people would agree that moving to a larger home in a better neighborhood is a good thing, but it is still stressful. We are used to living with chronic pain and suffering. Like the old home we decided to give up, it is where we are used to living. We became accustomed to feeling sick and being treated as sick. There are many reasons why we might not want to leave our old home. And there are many reasons why we might want to continue to be ill. Psychologists call this the sick role.

Some of us may have an unconscious desire to stay sick. That is to say, while we tell ourselves, our families, and our doctors that we want to get better, we are in conflict because part of us is used to being sick and acting sick. This may seem like a silly notion. "Who would want to stay sick?" we ask. "Certainly not I!" we say to ourselves. The fact is that some of us would rather continue to be sick than experience the fear or stress that accompanies change.

Some of us have not received much positive attention in our lives, so we might have grown needy and craving of attention. We have all heard of children who act out and disrupt the classroom to get attention. Could it be that, like the child who acts out, we, too, might also be getting attention in the wrong way? Since we are sick and in pain, we receive attention from family, friends, and healthcare professionals. We all need attention and companionship. There is nothing wrong with spending time with those who care for us. But there is a right way and a wrong way to get attention. If we have become comfortable with the sick role because it helps us get attention, then it is time to change. We will need to give up the sick role in order to overcome our suffering and develop healthy relationships.

Fear of failure is another reason for accepting things as they are rather than taking a risk. We may want very badly to succeed in our careers. We may want others to recognize our accomplishments. Our fear of failure may have kept us from taking risks so we did not reach our goals. It is normal to feel apprehensive about accepting a new job with bigger responsibilities. Part of us really wants that new job and all of the goodies that go with it; but the new job may involve spending time away from loved ones or taking on more responsibility than we want. We need to make decisions based on facts, not fear. If we use our medical problems as an excuse for not accepting challenges, we have chosen the sick role.

We are more dependent on others when we are ill. Some of us might have dependent personalities and have a strong need for others to help us manage. If we grew up in homes where there was a lot of chaos, we may crave the attention, affection, and security we did not receive as children. Those of us who have dependent personalities are afraid to face life's struggles alone. Since the sick role keeps us dependent on other people, fear of independence may be an unconscious reason to stay sick. But the sick role keeps us emotionally stuck, unable to move forward toward independence. Unconsciously wanting to stay sick, we magnify our pain.

To some extent, we have all adopted the sick role. Part of us wants to overcome our suffering and learn to interact with others in healthier ways. Part of us is more comfortable keeping things the way they are. We need to become healthier and more independent. In order to change, we must identify the obstacles that we have placed in our path of recovery. We will need to give up the sick role so we can deal effectively with life's challenges.

Adjusting to Change

We often find ourselves magnifying the importance of events in our lives. When faced with change, we spend too much time dwelling on the negative possibilities. Because bad things have happened to us in the past, we fear bad things will likely happen again. But this is not true. It is what psychologists call projection. We project our feelings into situations rather than being objective. There is an often-told ancient Chinese folk tale that teaches that things are not as they appear. The tale goes something like this:

There was once a wise old farmer who had lived with his only son. They had a small farm, and they needed their workhorse to plow the fields. One day, the farmer found that his horse had left through a broken fence.

When the friends of the old farmer heard about his horse running away, they tried to console him, and the wise farmer said, "How do you know this isn't good luck that my horse ran away?"

Several months later, the lost horse came back accompanied by a mare. He had found a mate! This time his friends were happy that the farmer was so lucky as to have two good horses. And the farmer said, "How do you know this isn't bad luck?"

When the old man's son fell off one of the horses and broke his leg, his neighbors came by to express their grief at this misfortune. He replied, "How do you know it isn't good luck that he fell from the horse?"

As the story goes, shortly after the man's son broke his leg, the emperor's army marched by the farm, taking away all able-bodied young men to fight a war against the Mongols. The farmer's son stayed on the farm. Was this good luck or bad luck?

Many of us look at adversity as catastrophes. We only see the bad. We do not to see the opportunities that arise from adversity. If we learn to accept today's misfortunes as a potential blessing for tomorrow, we might approach life's challenges with an attitude of positive expectancy instead of doom and gloom, and we would suffer less.

Fear of Abandonment

Some of us have lost some physical abilities, our independence, or our jobs as a result of our medical conditions. We may be unable to participate in social activities we once enjoyed. We may be less interested in sex, or no longer find it enjoyable. For these and many other reasons, we may feel increasingly vulnerable and afraid that family or friends may abandon us.

Fear of abandonment is normal for children. Children are dependent on their parents—needing them to provide shelter, food, safety, nurturing, and love. From a very early age, children learn to deal with situations when their needs are not met immediately. When a baby cries because she is hungry, she learns that she will be fed. With time, she cries less as she comes to expect regular feeding. Toddlers find the peek-a-boo game very amusing, but they are also learning an important lesson when they play this game; when the toddler's mother hides for a moment, the toddler feels apprehensive. The next second the child squeals with laughter at the release of tension and surprise of seeing her mother's face. The toddler playing peek-a-boo is not just having fun; she is learning trust. A child lost in a department store and separated from her mother for only a few minutes will often panic; this child may be fearful and clingy for days after the episode and need more attention than usual from the mother. Again, with time, the child learns to trust that her mother will take care of her.

Because of our medical conditions, we may be more dependent on others. This dependency may have brought back childhood insecurities and fears. It is important to recognize our emotions for what they are—just feelings. We may feel vulnerable, but that does not make us vulnerable. We are no longer children. We can learn to deal with our feelings in a mature, adult manner.

Distinguishing Needs from Wants

It is important for children to learn that their needs will be met. However, needs and wants are not the same, and all too often parents confuse the two. As an example, children rarely want to do homework; they would rather watch TV or play video games. But it is important for parents of grade school children to set aside homework time and review their homework assignments. When parents supervise homework, they are teaching scheduling, discipline, and other skills that children will need if they are to become successful, independent adults. They are also helping children to distinguish needs from wants.

Adults too have needs, and like children may confuse needs with wants. We all need food, shelter, safety, loving relationships, and activities that give us pleasure. Because of our situations, we may no longer be able to afford all of the "things" we want. We may no longer be able to engage in the activities we enjoy. If we are unable to distinguish our wants from needs, we may find ourselves bitter and frustrated.

Dealing with Frustration

All children learn to deal with frustration, but some better than others. Our childhood helps shape our temperament and our ability to adjust to change. When faced with adversity, some of us are able to remain calm and positive, while others are not. Under stress, we all tend to revert to habits we learned as children. How do children learn to cope with frustration? How well did we learn? Can we develop new coping skills?

Anyone who has been a parent knows that toddlers have problems at bedtime. Because children need sleep, parents put them to bed, even though the toddler may want to stay up and play. Temper tantrums often result. There are different ways of handling this common problem—some better than others. One way would be to pick up the crying child immediately, but parents soon learn that this is not a very effective strategy, because the child screams again shortly after the parent leaves the room. Sometimes parents respond inconsistently to crying, one time with immediate attention and at other times letting the child cry for a long time. Children treated in this way will not know what to expect, and the bedtime crying episodes tend to increase in duration; psychologists call this "intermittent reinforcement"—a surefire way to reinforce and maintain a bad behavior. Pediatricians recommend that parents take a systematic approach to bedtime crying, coming into the bedroom at increasing time intervals to reassure the child of their presence, but not picking up the child. In this way, children learn to comfort themselves—an important life skill. When we cannot get what we want, do we still bang our fists on our cribs? Are we frustrated, angry, irritable or demanding? Do we wonder why our loved ones sometimes respond to our needs and sometimes don't? If so, it is time to make a change. We need to learn to distinguish needs from wants and to take better care of ourselves.

We Need Each Other

Many of us have used ineffective coping strategies to deal with our fears, insecurities, and our pain. We might have spent too much time worrying, because worry makes us believe we could control life's circumstances by thinking about all the possibilities—but it really accomplishes little or nothing other than to make us crazy. We may have become compulsively self-reliant so that we never have to risk rejection. Some of us never learned to recognize our own needs, so we spend too much time trying to please others. This just adds to stress, and stress increases pain.

We began our Twelve Step program by recognizing that we cannot control the fact that we are in pain, and that we need to develop a relationship with a Higher Power in order to overcome our suffering. Belief in a Higher Power is important to recovery. Through this belief, we come to understand it is our duty to find purpose in life. In the past, we may have made choices to seek the approval of family or friends rather than to meet our own needs. Guided by our Higher Power, we will make better decisions. As we learn to trust in the Higher Power, our fear will melt away. Since fear plays such an important role in our suffering, overcoming fear is a major step in our recovery.

No one can work a Twelve-Step program alone. No one can recover from suffering without the help of others. Humans are social beings. We need each other to live. From the time we are born, we need love and nurturing. An infant denied the physical comfort of human touch but provided with a crib, infant formula, a warm room, and regular diaper change will fail to grow and may eventually die; doctors call this syndrome "failure to thrive." Sadly, children deprived of touch sometimes become so sick that they are admitted into the hospital where nurses or volunteers hold, comfort, and speak to them; these babies begin to gain weight almost immediately. Humans are social creatures and we need the help of family, friends, teachers, coaches, and many others to live happy, healthy lives.

Just as children need care, attention and love, so too do adults. To fulfill our purpose, we need to identify our real needs and ask others to help us. We need to learn who is willing and able. If we fail to ask for help, or choose the wrong people to trust, we will be saddled with unmet physical and emotional needs. This will only increase our suffering.

Intimacy—Real Relationships

When psychologists talk about intimacy, they are not talking about sex. Sex can be part of an intimate relationship, but it is not the only part. An intimate relationship is one where there is honest, trusting communication between two people who want to help each other. In order to recover from our suffering, we need intimate relationships. Honesty is the first step toward intimacy. First, we must be honest with ourselves. This is why we made a list of our strengths and weaknesses. Next, we must place our trust in another person, so we can share the facts of our lives, especially our vulnerabilities and weaknesses.

Intimate relationships are not easy to develop or maintain. If we are not used to honest sharing, we need to find someone we know we can trust. We need to know that this person will be responsive to our needs, keep our confidence, and be neutral and non-judgmental. This person must also understand that emotional and spiritual suffering makes our physical pain worse. This may be a friend or family member, but it is often easier to trust a therapist, member of the clergy, or a Twelve Step sponsor.

Intimate relationships mean truly sharing ourselves with others. Intimate relationships mean that each person commits to help the other—avoiding all manipulation or "using" one another. As we share our inventory for the first time, we will be sharing our pain and our suffering. In sharing our inventory, we commit to making our lives meaningful—both personally and spiritually. It is an honor to be chosen to listen to someone share a personal inventory. It is also a gift. The process of sharing helps both parties develop a greater connection to each other, and, in the process, improve their conscious connection with the Higher Power. It is through honest sharing that we experience the healing power of love. Honest sharing is part of the Higher Power's plan for us—it brings truth from falsehood, light from darkness, and peace from conflict.

Inspirational Reading—Auguste Renoir

"The pain passes, but the beauty remains."

"The work of art must seize upon you, wrap you up in itself, and carry you away. It is the means by which the artist conveys his passion. It is the current which he puts forth, which sweeps you along in his passion."

Auguste Renoir was born in 1841. Although trained in traditional art and porcelain painting, he often experimented with new art forms. Even among other artists, he had an extraordinary ability to blend colors—needing only five colors on his palette to create any shade he wished. He was one of the first to adopt the impressionist painting style, and is now recognized as one the founders of the impressionist movement. Prints of his paintings are found in homes and museums throughout the world—a statement to the enduring popularity of his work.

Although millions of people are familiar with Renoir's work, most are unaware that he suffered from debilitating arthritis in his later years. Renoir did not let painful arthritis deter him from his painting. He continued to paint when others would have given up. Toward the end of his life, he would tie artist brushes to his deformed hands so that he could continue to paint. Nothing could deter him from his purpose.

Can you imagine being an artist with crippled hands? Overcoming the pain of severe arthritis required positive feelings and beliefs; Renoir could not see a future that did not allow him to create works of art. He did not see arthritis as an insurmountable barrier. He did not spend time wallowing in self-pity or defeatism. Renoir knew that he was meant to create art, and he overcame whatever obstacles life placed in his way.

Prayer for the Fifth Step

My inventory has shown me who I am. I ask for help in admitting my shortcomings. Give me the courage to share them with another person. I pray for guidance in this step, so that I can honestly share the facts of my life with another.

Exercise for the Fifth Step

Obstacles to Trust:

Real relationships require honest sharing. We need to honestly address why we may be reluctant to share ourselves with others. In this exercise, choose the one or more adults who are most important in your life. In considering these relationships, answer the following questions:

-What things about yourself that are you most afraid to share? (Remember, the things that bother you the most are probably the very things you need to share.)

-Are you jealous when they receive attention from others?

-Do you find yourself saying what you think they might want to hear, but not what you really believe?

-Do you overreact to their criticism?

-Are you afraid that if they really knew you, they would think less of you?

-Do you tend to lose yourself in these relationships, becoming more concerned with their problems than your own?

-Do you abandon your own interests to conform to theirs?

After answering these questions, you must decide whether any of the people you chose should hear your inventory. It is precisely because many of us have problems in relationships that Twelve Step programs recommend sharing with a therapist, sponsor, or clergy. With time, you will strengthen your relationships with those closest to you and begin to share more of yourself with them.

Chapter 6

Letting Love Heal our Wounds

Chronic Pain Step 6: Were entirely ready to have our Higher Power remove all these defects of character.

Nicole's Story

"My back pain started when I was thirty years old. I am a nurse, and it isn't uncommon for nurses to have back problems. We often find ourselves bending over hospital beds to lift patients. My doctor prescribed oxycodone for pain, and it allowed me to continue working. I began needing more and more medication, and found that I couldn't stop. When I became pregnant, I had to tell my obstetrician that I was on opioids for pain, and he admitted me to the hospital. The doctors diagnosed me as being addicted and began methadone—a standard treatment for pregnant women who are addicted. I had never been addicted to anything in my life! I don't smoke. I hardly ever drank. I never used drugs. I was married, working, and have children. I couldn't believe this had happened to me. A few months into my pregnancy, I was admitted to the hospital with bleeding. I lost my baby. I thought this was entirely my fault.

My physician called in an addiction specialist. The specialist explained that I had lost control of my opioid use, and that I was using them for reasons other than for pain relief. I had to admit that this was true. I found that oxycodone gave me energy and relaxed me. I also had to admit that I had had problems with anxiety, self-esteem, and trust for as long as I could remember.

I grew up in a poor family. As the oldest child, I had to help my parents care for my younger brothers and sisters. Because we lived in a rough neighborhood, my parents kept me from playing with the children on the block. I tried hard to cover-up my insecurities through achievement. I was the first person in my family to go to college. I was also the first to escape poverty. However, I was not the first to feel insecure.

It has been a year since I got honest with my husband, my doctor, and myself. I am now off pain medications. I have found better ways of coping with life's stresses. I am very involved with my family and my church. I learned that I do not have to take care of others to feel good about myself. I have learned to ask for help when I need it. I have learned that each day is a blessing!"

Letting Love Heal Our Wounds

Culture and technology have shaped spiritual beliefs and practices since humans first walked upon the earth. Until the coming of the industrial age, seasonal agricultural labor played an important role in most people's lives. They worked hard during planting and harvest times, paying close attention to seasonal changes, weather conditions, and other factors thought to influence crop production and reproductive cycles. The wheel of life turns season-by-season, year-by-year. As our ancestors did before us, we celebrate holidays to mark the changing seasons. Spring is a time of awakening and rebirth—when animals give birth to their young, plants emerge from the soil, and trees first stir from their winter rest. It is also a time for spiritual rebirth. Christians celebrate Easter at the first full moon after the spring equinox—the date when daytime and nighttime are equal in length. The word Easter itself comes from the name of a goddess of spring—Eostre.

The early Christian Church chose dates for its holidays to coincide with important dates in the pagan calendar. As an example, it recognized a day close to the fall equinox as the hallowed eve before the feast of All Saints. Ancient pagan peoples thought spirits roamed the earth after nightfall; the fall equinox marked the time when nights would become longer than days, so the spirits would became more powerful. Today, children celebrate Halloween—dressing up as goblins and ghosts, mostly unaware that beliefs about saints and the spirit world gave rise to this holiday.

For the ancient Germanic peoples, groves of fir trees were sacred places. Since Christians did not know the exact time of year when Christ was born, early church leaders chose a time near the winter solstice to celebrate the holiday, and marked this holiday by bringing fir trees into their homes as Christmas trees.

Before the industrial age, people relied on open fires and oil lamps for lighting. They were much more aware of weather, seasons, and nature in general than we are. Families gathered for evening meals at dusk. Often, they prayed before each meal, giving thanks for the blessings that had brought food to the table. The industrial revolution has forever changed our relationships with nature and other people. Modern conveniences made possible extended work hours, shift work, business travel, and after-dark recreational activities. For many of us, it is no longer possible to plan family meals because everyone is so busy. Millions of us now eat at fast food restaurants, where it is unusual to see customers with heads bowed in pre-hamburger prayer. Family function has changed significant as a result of modern lifestyles..

Of course, change is inevitable, and we must adapt, but that does not mean we must leave behind our traditions and spiritual beliefs. It has become increasingly difficult to find time for the spiritual in our daily lives. In our modern society, religious worship is less important than it was for our ancestors. Many of us now limit worship to attendance at weddings, funerals, and major holidays, such as Christmas, Easter, Passover, or Yom Kippur. There are exceptions, of course. Observant Muslims kneel and pray at appointed times each day, and fast for the entire month of Ramadan. Orthodox Jews strictly observe Sabbath as a day of rest and prayer and many will not drive a car or answer the telephone on this day. Catholics and other Christians may observe the Lenten fast and attend services regularly in the weeks before Easter. However, for many of us religious worship is now the exception, not the rule. Religion is often an afterthought in this media-driven society where manufacturing, marketing, and selling consumer goods are of paramount importance. We believe that there is a Higher Power, that there is right and wrong, and that we are part of the Higher Power's plan, but we often skimp on time to connect with the Higher Power. How then do we make room for the spiritual and the sacred in our lives?

Lessons from Sacred Books

There is a tradition in many cultures of using stories, myths, or parables to teach about our relationship with the Higher Power. We often fail to recognize the sacred and divine in our busy lives. This was also true in ancient times. In the Gospel of Luke (24:13-35), two travelers were walking along the road to Emmaus. They were lamenting the recent death of Jesus—their spiritual leader. As they were walking, the resurrected Jesus arrived and joined in the conversation. Thinking Jesus dead, they did not recognize him. Later that day, they came to stop at a tavern where Jesus joined them for dinner. He broke bread and poured wine as he did at the Last Supper and only then were "their eyes opened" to the presence of the divine in their midst. According the Gospel, Jesus then vanished from their sight.

In Genesis (18:1-15), Abraham and his wife Sarah entertained three strangers in their home. They made bread and slaughtered a lamb to honor their guests. The three guests turned out to be angels. The angels ate and then announced that Sarah would bear a son. In another Genesis story (19:1-11), Lot entertained two strangers, prepared a meal for them and offered them shelter. When villagers tried to break down Lot's door to attack the strangers, the two strangers revealed themselves as angels and struck the attackers blind so they were unable to find the door.

Stories such as these teach that us even the just and righteous often fail to recognize the presence of a Higher Power in their lives. This is part of the human condition. We are often too concerned with our daily activities to attend to our spiritual needs.

Must We Be So Busy?

Modern conveniences free us from the drudgery of work, but we seem to be busier than ever. Some of us work two jobs to make ends meet. We skip family dinners so we can spend time at the gym. We try to schedule quality time with our families, but this is easier said than done. We settle instead for text messages and Facebook posts. If life seems like a crazy, spinning carousel, it may be time to step off! We may need to reorder our priorities and make time for prayer or meditation.

We may need to ask ourselves if we really must be so busy. For some of us, the answer is "no." We may have fallen into the trap created by modern commercial enterprise. We may be working extra hard to buy things we want, but do not need. We may be working to keep up with our neighbors. Companies are in the business of selling products or services, and their advertisements entice us to believe that our lives will be better if we buy them. But is this really true? Do we really need a new car, more expensive athletic shoes, a bigger TV, vitamin enriched water, or the latest fashion clothing? We may spend hours on end looking at catalogs or surfing the Internet for things to buy—time we could use attending to real needs. We must ask ourselves if we are sacrificing time that we should be spending with family and friends or attending to our spiritual needs. What would our lives be like if we paid less attention to the advertising hype?

Are Others Really Living the Good Life?

Because of our injuries or medical conditions, we may feel that we are less fortunate than others are. We may be resentful of those who are wealthier, in better health, or more physically attractive than we are. Bitterness and resentment often follow losses of any kind, but especially the loss of function that accompanies painful medical conditions. We need to look past the superficial appearances of happiness and success. A popular bumper sticker says, "He who dies with the most toys wins the game." Do we really believe this is true? Most of us would agree that there is more truth in the saying, "When the chess game is over, the king and the pawns go back in the same box."

We all know of celebrities who seemed to have had it all— wealth, fame, beauty, and physical health, only to turn to drugs or commit suicide. In reality, these individual may have been missing out on the most important things in life. When we are honest with ourselves, we know that happiness requires adequate food, shelter, clothing, and health—but how much more? Once our basic needs are met, more stuff rarely brings happiness. If scientists were to have invented both a happiness meter and a time machine, and if we took that happiness meter back in time 50 years, how much less happiness would it register than today? Some might argue that the meter might show more happiness because marketing creates false needs that cannot be met. Some might argue that we are less happy because we must work so hard to buy consumer goods. Real happiness comes from satisfying relationships, achieving our potential, and having a connection with something greater than ourselves. Resentment of other people's apparent good fortune or our bad fortune just keeps us stuck in the past and distracts us from the work we must do, if we are to find peace and happiness in our lives.

Changing our Beliefs about Ourselves

We all have beliefs, but some beliefs are more important to us than are others. Some beliefs are easy to change but others are not. We do not get particularly upset when we find out that we were fooled into believing in an "urban legend" (don't alligators live in New York City sewers?). On the other hand, some beliefs are very difficult to change. Some beliefs, such as religious faith beliefs, are so strong that we call them convictions. Our beliefs profoundly affect how we experience pain. We need to identify those beliefs that may contribute to our suffering, and decide whether we can change them. Some will be easier to change than others.

Building on the Work of Our Ancestors

All cultures have traditions, holidays, or religious practices that remind group members to be grateful for the contributions of ancestors. In some cultures, individuals trace their lineage to a god, to a divinely inspired person or event. The sacred texts of the Jewish, Christian, and Islamic faiths refer to Abraham as the father of a chosen people, and describe the lives of Abraham's offspring and successive generations. Some religions encourage the practice of ancestor worship, venerating deceased whom they believe are living spirits who remain part of the family. Other religions emphasize the contributions of enlightened teachers, saints, or martyrs to their faith. National holidays remind us of the contributions of others to country, national heritage, and daily lives. Some of us seek to learn more about our lineage by conducting online genealogy searches or having DNA analyzed to trace ethnicity. By connecting to our past, we may be able to overcome our sense of isolation and increase awareness of our interdependence.

Most of us recognize our indebtedness to past generations, but those of us who grew up in abusive households may be angry with our parents; it may be hard for them to believe that ancestors are important let alone worthy of worship. When we consider ourselves as the ancestors of future generations, we begin to understand the importance of our own place in history. We realize that each successive generation builds on the work of proceeding generations. Our parents, for all of their shortcomings, may have done a better job in raising us than their parents did in raising them. When our parents' best was not good enough, it leaves us with emotional wounds that add to our physical pain. We need to understand that our parents may also have had deep emotional wounds. They may have been angry with their own parents, and our children may be angry with us. It is our job to make the world a better place

92

for the succeeding generations. By working our Twelve Step recovery program, we build upon the work of those who came before us, and we strengthen the foundation for future generations.

Inspirational Reading—Joni Eareckson Tada

"God deliberately chooses weak, suffering and unlikely candidates to get His work done, so that in the end, the glory goes to God and not to the person."

"Wait on the Lord in prayer as you sit on the freeway, sharing with him the anxiety of so many jobs to be done in such a short time. Watch your frustrations melt into praise as you sing hymns and choruses for his ears alone."

"When we suffer and handle it with grace, we are like walking billboards advertising the way God works in the life of someone who suffers"

Joni Eareckson was born in Baltimore. She was an active young woman who enjoyed tennis, camping, swimming, and horseback riding. She graduated high school in 1967. A few weeks later, on a hot July day, Joni met her sister and some friends at a Chesapeake Bay beach. Shortly after arriving at the beach, she dove into the water striking the bottom with her head. She immediately knew something was wrong because she could not move her legs. Her sister and friends saved her from drowning.

Once a vigorous, athletic woman, Joni Eareckson was now a quadriplegic. While her friends were busy preparing to go to college in the fall, Joni was confined to a wheelchair, learning to accept the fact that she would never walk again. For a period of time, Joni was depressed. Her life had seemingly lost its meaning. She could not understand how God could let this happen to her. Through her prayers and through the love of family and friends, Joni's depression gradually lifted. She came to believe that everything in life has a reason, including her diving accident.

During her physical rehabilitation, Joni learned to paint detailed pictures using a brush that she held between her teeth. Her paintings were of such high quality that collectors bought them. Because of her remarkable achievements, she became widely known and was invited to appear on television programs. Painting was just the beginning of Joni Eareckson's new life. Joni discovered that she would soon play a special role in advocating for others with disabilities. She became a bestselling author, an inspirational speaker, and a talk show radio host. Her books have been translated into fifteen languages, and she has traveled to more than thirty countries spreading her message of hope and love. She also served on the National Council on Disability. Joni and Friends—the nonprofit organization she founded in 1979—provides services for thousands of disabled individuals throughout the world.

Joni Eareckson would never consider someone with disabilities to be any less a person than those who appears to be in good health. In fact, she sees a special role for those who suffer. She draws her message of hope from the Christian Bible. In the Gospel stories, Christ ministers to the weak, the poor, and the sick. He taught that those so afflicted were actually closer to God than the rich and the fortunate. "How can this be?" many of us may ask. For Joni Eareckson the message was quite clear. Those who appear so well off often have little reason to challenge their beliefs about themselves or the world around them; it is easier for them to go about their lives without ever awakening to reality. In contrast, those who have had to suffer may be more likely to be honest in their self-appraisal, more accepting of their weaknesses, more likely to be grateful for life's blessings, more empathetic to others, and more open to the Higher Power that sustains us all.

Today, many receive healthcare from institutions with the word "Samaritan" in their names. . Samaritans played a special role in the *Bible*. In one story, a man lies beaten at the side of the road. Many passed him by without offering help, but a Samaritan came to his aid. The story has meaning for us when we realize that most Jews scorned Samaritans as a second-class, mixed race that did not follow the Temple rules. It was precisely because the "good Samaritan" had known suffering that he had empathy for the man at the side of the road. Today, if we try to help someone on the side of the road, Good Samaritan laws protect us from lawsuits. Joni Eareckson teaches us that we, too, can find strength in our pain. We, too, can be good Samaritans.

Prayer for the Sixth Step

I pray for help to continue being honest with myself so that I will be ready to receive the guidance I need to remove my defects in character. Guide me toward spiritual and mental health.

Exercise for the Sixth Step

Many of us believe things that are not true (such as the urban legend about alligators in the New York sewers). We need to discover whether negative beliefs hinder our recovery. Answer each of the questions below:

-Do you believe that there is no future for yourself? Or do you see a positive future?

-Do you believe that you are not worthwhile? Or that you have an important role to play in the lives of others?

-Do you believe that you are not a whole person because of pain or disability? Or do you believe that you are no less a person because you have a painful condition?

-Do you believe that if you can no longer do all the things you used to do, life is not worthwhile? Or that there are many meaningful things you can still do?

-Do you believe that pain makes you a weak person? Or do you believe that pain makes you stronger?

-Do you believe that you will always be pain-ridden? Or can you see a day when your pain level will be acceptable?

In answering these questions, consider the following:

-Why do you believe the things you do?

-Did you learn negative thinking from others?

-How did your parents handle adversity?

-How many of your negative beliefs are rooted in low self-esteem or shame?

-What facts would make you change your mind about your beliefs?

-What would happen to you if you gave up these beliefs?

Chapter 7

Letting Go of Our Pride

Chronic Pain Step 7: Humbly asked our Higher Power for the strength to overcome our shortcomings, so that we can carry out the Higher Power's will for us.

Robert's Story

"I am a 44-year-old, successful businessman who is married with three children. My life was great until I developed low back pain about two years ago. I don't recall any specific injury. I just began having more and more pain. I ended up seeing my family doctor, then an orthopedic specialist, and finally a pain specialist at a well-known medical school. I was told I had bulging discs in my lumbar spine. They treated me with spinal injections, OxyContin ® and Percocet ®. My pain continued, and I needed more medication. One day, I called the specialist for more pain medication. He wouldn't refill my prescription because they said it was too early. They were treating me like I was an addict. I was really upset and called my family doctor. He sent me to another specialist.

The new specialist was very interested in my past. I explained to him that I was a lucky individual, up until my back pain. I was raised in a great family. I had no problems growing up. After college, I joined my father in running the family business. I married a wonderful woman and we have great kids. Back pain changed everything.

After a few sessions with the specialist, I came to realize that back pain was just one of reasons I was suffering. I didn't want to admit it, but I wasn't really happy working in my family business. I was resentful about things that happened at work. I was isolating myself from my wife and our children. I found it hard to let people know that I had problems and that I needed their help. I had to overcome my pride.

I made a lot of progress within a few months, but it has been hard work. I realized that my back pain began when I took on more responsibility at work and I was afraid of failure. Oxycodone did more than relieve my pain; it also gave me energy and confidence. I was using a narcotic to manage my emotions. On a few occasions, the pain specialist asked my wife to come to his office with me. I came to realize that part of my recovery was improving our relationship. I learned that pride had kept me from admitting that I needed help.

Letting Go of Our Pride

The English word "pride" has many connotations. It may mean getting pleasure from doing something well—as in taking pride in one's work. We tell our children that we are proud when we praise their accomplishments. But pride can also mean having an inflated sense of self worth. In the classic Greek tragedies of the fourth century BCE, the main character was a hero who, like all of us, had strengths and weaknesses. More often than not, one of these weaknesses was hubris—the Greek word for pride, and the hero ultimately suffered a great loss because of this tragic character flaw. Although Greek tragedies were written over 2,000 years ago, literature, drama and film students still study them, because the theme of the flawed hero appeals to audiences today as well as it did to the ancient Greeks. We all have heroes—political figures, actors, sports stars, and singers. None of them is perfect. There is something very reassuring when they mess up.

Pete Rose was an American baseball player whose exceptional performance guaranteed that he would become a member of the Baseball Hall of Fame. In 1975, he was named "Sportsman of the Year" by *Sports Illustrated* magazine. But it was later learned that Pete Rose placed bets on professional baseball games—something that is strictly forbidden by Major League Baseball. Though his athletic performance certainly merited induction into baseball's Hall of Fame, he has been denied that honor for many years, not so much because he bet on baseball, but because he steadfastly refused to admit it. His stubborn pride tarnished his reputation and his standing as a celebrity. Pete Rose is a tragic hero whose life became the subject of the movie *Hustle*—a modern day tragedy. We can learn a lesson from the life of Pete Rose. Setting aside our pride is a hard, but necessary part of our recovery.

The problem for many of us is distinguishing healthy self-esteem from an inflated sense of self-worth. We all need self-esteem. Each of us is worthwhile and deserving of respect, dignity, and love. Pride is not the same as self-esteem. We can have low self-esteem and be prideful. In fact, low self-esteem can cause us to become overly proud or arrogant. We may try to overcome low self-esteem by telling ourselves that wealth or social standing makes us better than others. We may feel we need to criticize others in order to make us feel good about ourselves. Our misguided efforts to boost our self-esteem at the expense of others will only cause more suffering. How can we overcome our pride?

Prayer requires us to be honest with ourselves. It requires us to be humble—to have a balanced understanding of both our strengths and our weaknesses. We should be thankful for

99

our strengths, and pray to overcome our weaknesses. Prayer should not be a "wish list" of material things that we believe would make us feel better. When some of us were children, we might have made lists of toys we wanted from Santa Claus for Christmas, but as we grew older, we came to realize this holiday is giving to other in order to express love and appreciation.

Humility means that we fairly assess our strengths and our weaknesses, not taking credit for the work of others or the work of the Higher Power in our lives. No one is successful without the help of others, and our very lives depend on a Power greater than ourselves. When we judge ourselves superior or more deserving than others, we disconnect ourselves from those around us. Humility necessitates owning up to our mistakes, and correcting them. Pride keeps us from accepting responsibility by blaming others so that we can look or feel good at their expense. Humility gives us an honest perspective of our true role in society.

Pride keeps us from honestly assessing our own strengths and weaknesses. The Nazi party in Germany based itself on false pride. Followers took pride in watching SS troops march in parades. They took pride in new weaponry, grandiose new buildings, and, above all, in their mistaken belief that they belonged to a superior race. So strong was their pride in their party and their country that most Nazis continued to defend the party and its hideous actions even as their country was bombed into ruins. The Nazi movement was the quintessence of pride on an institutionalization level, and it culminated in the death of millions of innocents. Many wars have been waged because of national pride. Many more will follow. No one benefits from this kind of pride. Peacemakers honestly assess their own strengths and weakness, seek to understand the positions of opposing sides, and try to avoid conflict by emphasizing those things that bind people together rather than keep them apart.

100

When we find ourselves criticizing others, we must look at our own motives. Are we judging other people, or are we judging their actions? Are our criticisms justified? Are we falling into the trap of criticizing others in order to feel better about ourselves?

In this step, we humbly seek strength from the Higher Power so that we can overcome our shortcomings. We cannot proceed without honestly looking at our pride. Pride is present in all of us. We need to set it aside in order to achieve humility—the honest assessment of our strengths and weaknesses.

Inspirational Reading – A Psalm of David

Lord, do not rebuke me in your anger, or discipline me in your wrath. For your arrows have sunk into me, and your hand has come down on me. There is no soundness in my flesh because of your indignation; there is no health in my bones because of my sin. For my iniquities have gone over my head; they weigh like a burden too heavy for me. My wounds grow foul and fester because of my foolishness; I am utterly bowed down and prostrate; all day long I go around mourning. For my loins are filled with burning, and there is no soundness in my flesh. I am utterly spent and crushed; I groan because of the tumult of my heart fails me; as for the light of my eyes—it also has gone from me...

But it is for you, O Lord, that I wait; it is you, O Lord my God, who will answer. For I pray, "Only do not let them rejoice over me, those who boast against me when my foot slips. "For I am ready to fall, and my pain is ever with me. I confess my iniquity; I am sorry for my sin. Those who are my foes without cause are mighty, and many are those who hate me wrongfully. Those who render me evil for good are my adversaries

101

because I follow after good. Do not forsake me, O Lord; O my God, do not be far from me ;make haste to help me, O Lord, my salvation.

Christians and Jews are familiar with the *Bible* story of David and Goliath. David was a young shepherd boy who, armed only with a sling and stone shot, faced and vanquished the mighty Philistine warrior Goliath in battle. David went on to become one of the most famous kings of the Israelites but one who also succumbed to temptations. The *Bible* describes how David came to have an affair with a married woman, Bathsheba. When Bathsheba became pregnant, David sent her husband off to the front lines of a war knowing full well that he would be killed. David then brought Bathsheba to his palace to become one of his wives. The prophet Nathan confronted David over his infidelity, deceit and murder of Bathsheba's husband and David repented his sins.

David, the author or editor of many of the psalms, lived to old age and suffered from both physical illness and emotional pain. David went from being the conquering hero of the Israelites to a King who struggled mightily with his own weaknesses. The excerpt above from Psalm 38, David expresses his belief that God is the source of healing, and that suffering comes from our own words and deeds. This is a psalm of penitence in which David admits his wrongdoings, admits his powerlessness to change the opinion of others, and asks God for forgiveness and healing. David humbles himself before God, because he knows he must give up his pride in order to be healed. At one point, David had felt close to God, but greed and power corrupted him. In this psalm, he prays for a closer connection with God.

As it was for David over 2,000 years ago, it is still true that we have made mistakes and have suffered the consequences. Like David, we must humble ourselves. In honestly assessing our strengths and weaknesses, we make room in our lives for the Higher Power to heal us.

Prayer for the Seventh Step

I have admitted my faults. With humility and openness I seek to eliminate our shortcomings. I pray now for daily progress in overcoming my defects in character. Grant me strength, so I can do so.

Exercise for the Seventh Step

In this exercise, we look for false pride in ourselves and humbly ask the Higher Power to remove this shortcoming. Without humility, we cannot have recovery. We must be committed to an honest assessment of ourselves. Only in this way can we overcome isolation and connect with others.

-Do you feel that you are better than others because you belong to a certain group?

-Do you feel that you are better than others because you have endured pain?

-Do you feel that you are better than others because you pray often or attend worship services?

-Do you feel that you are better than others because you of your social status?

If you answered, "yes" to these questions, you must accept the fact that you have bolstered your self-esteem at the expense of humility. When you come to understand that your self-worth does not come from others, but from the Higher Power, you will start to overcome false pride.

Chapter 8

Accepting Responsibility for Our Deeds

Chronic Pain Step 8: Made a list of all the persons we had harmed because we were controlled by our pain and our fear, and became willing to make amends to them all.

Mark's Story

"I am a 40-year-old man who has suffered from chronic back pain for years. I had gone to orthopedic and pain specialists, but no treatment was very successful. Because my job involves physical work, I missed a lot of time. I asked for 'light duty' assignments, but these were hard to get. Finally, my boss told me that he would have to lay me off because I missed so much time. This made me really angry. I wanted to work, but I was in pain. Without a job I felt useless. My wife had to work overtime to help make ends meet. I felt that I was no longer a real man. I was angry because I had gotten such a rotten deal. I was angry with my boss for letting me go. Sometimes, I was angry with my wife because she had little time for me. We argued a lot about money. I spent less time with my friends. Often I had a short fuse with my kids. I wanted the support and understanding from my family and when I didn't get what I thought I deserved, I got even angrier. I was afraid I would never get a new job. I was afraid about what others would think of me. I was in pain and I was miserable.

Eventually, I came to understand that my emotions played a big role in my pain. I brought my wife to one of the doctor visits so he could explain this to her. During that office visit, both my wife and I talked about our feelings. I told her that I was sorry for being so angry and irritable. I promised to make it up to her.

Now my pain is manageable. I have made a lot of progress in my recovery. I am back to work in a less stressful job. I accept the fact that I used to blame my bad behavior on my pain. Pain was a poor excuse for my bitterness, resentment, and isolation. Along the way I have had to make amends to friends and family for neglecting my obligations."

Accepting Responsibility for Our Deeds

As hard as we try, we will never be able to make amends for all of our wrongdoings. In taking on the sick role, we harm ourselves and those closest to us. Making amends is important, but not as important as our willingness to do so. Willingness means we must be prepared to set aside our anger, resentment, and fear. Willingness requires a commitment to be honest with ourselves first, and then with others. Willingness means being ready to give up our negative beliefs and feelings. Since we learned that negativity causes suffering, we have little choice.

Inspirational Reading—Rumi

"Everyone has been made for some particular work, and the desire for that work has been put in every heart."

"It may be that the satisfaction I need depends on my going away, so that when I've gone and come back, I'll find it at home."

"Something opens our wings. Something makes boredom and hurt disappear. Someone fills the cup in front of us. We taste only sacredness. "

"The breeze at dawn has secrets to tell you; don't go back to sleep. You must ask for what you really want; don't go back to sleep. People are going back and forth across the doorsill where the two worlds touch. The door is round and open. Don't go back to sleep."

"The dark thought, the shame, the malice, meet them at your door laughing, and invite them in. Be grateful for whoever comes, because each has been sent as a guide from beyond."

Jalaluddin Rumi was born in 1207 in what is now Afghanistan. His family fled that region to avoid the Mongols who were expanding their territory under the Khan Empire. He traveled with his family to Baghdad and then on to the Moslem holy city of Mecca. Along the way, Rumi and his family endured many hardships traveling through the mountains and deserts of the Middle East. Eventually, they settled in what is now western Turkey, living among people known as the "Rum." Jalaluddin is known to us by the name Rumi, because he spent most of his life living in this region of Turkey.

Jalaluddin took up the study of the *Koran*—the holy book of Islam, and followed the family tradition of becoming a religious teacher. During his studies, he became familiar with Sufi teachings. The Sufis seek a mystical union with God; they see each person as having gifts that are manifestations of God. Sufis believe that we place obstacles in the way of true awareness: acting out of anger, gratifying addictions and other cravings, seeking fulfillment through material means. Sufi's

107

seek a mystical connection God through prayer, contemplation and meditation. Poetry was an important part of Rumi's mystical practice, and he composed over 30,000 versus of poetry. Rumi taught that Muslims, Christians, Jews, and Zoroastrians should be viewed as brethren. When Rumi died, men and women of many faiths are said to have pressed through a huge crowd to touch the green cloth that covered his coffin. Today, his mausoleum in Turkey is a place of pilgrimage for thousands. Rumi is recognized as one of the greatest poets of history, and his poetry can be found in bookstores throughout the world. He is perhaps the most read poet of all times, and readers find truth in his poetry many centuries after it was written.

Eighth Step Prayer

I ask for help in making a list of all those I have harmed. I will take responsibility for my mistakes and be forgiving to others as you are forgiving to me. Grant me the willingness to begin my restitution. This I pray.

Exercise for the Eight Step

Having already made a fearless inventory of our weaknesses, and having prayed for the courage to correct our wrongdoings, we are ready to make a list of those we have injured. In making this list, we must be entirely honest with ourselves.

It is important that each of us take responsibility for our own words and actions. Answer each of the questions below to the best of your ability. Remember, this exercise is part of your healing process. The questions below are not all inclusive; they serve as examples only.

-Have you caused others to feel guilty as a way of getting your needs met?

-Have you shirked your duties or failed to act responsibly using pain as an excuse?

-Have your relationships with loved ones suffered because you isolated yourself from them?

-Have you caused financial harm because you could have worked, but were wallowing in self-pity?

-Have you harmed your children's emotional development through neglect, abuse, or bad example?

-Have you blamed others for your problems and failed to take responsibility?

Chapter 9

Making Amends to Others and Ourselves

Chronic Pain Step 9: Made direct amends to such people wherever possible, except when to do so would injure them or others.

Vince's Story

"I am a 40-year-old professional. I first remember having problems with abdominal pain when I was in college. I would often have cramps and diarrhea, especially under stress. I also had bladder problems. When these conditions got bad enough, I went to see doctors who diagnosed me as having irritable bowel syndrome and chronic prostate inflammation. Medications helped some, but the problems continued. I decided to read about these conditions and found that many experts linked both of them to stress. This is not what I wanted to hear.

I am now on a road to recovery. I realize that as a child I was unhappy and frightened. I believed I was physically unattractive, I never wanted anyone to take my picture, and I avoided looking in mirrors. I had few friends. I a good student and went to college on a scholarship. Doing well in school seemed to boost my self-esteem. I graduated at the top of my college class and went on to graduate school. But even these successes didn't make me feel good about myself. I decided it was time to settle down, get married, and have children. It seemed okay for a while, but I continued to push myself. Within a few years, I had climbed to the top of the company where I worked, but my stomach cramps and bladder problems were worse than ever. I had to accept the fact that I was a workaholic and no amount of success would be good enough. I also had to accept the fact that I didn't spend enough time with my children, and often blamed my wife for my unhappiness.

I had to make amends in order to I get honest with myself and with my family. I had to own up to the fact that I was not the tough, successful professional I had pretended to be. I was a frightened, insecure man who was afraid of intimacy. I had to apologize for what I had done wrong and commit to overcoming my inadequacies. I still get adnominal cramps once in a while, but only when I am under a lot of stress. Now, I see a bright future."

Making Amends—Atonement

Making amends is a way of atoning for what we have done wrong. A man who stole his neighbor's power tools replaces them. A woman who lied to a friend apologizes and tells the truth. An employee who neglected his job responsibilities works harder than expected. Making amends can be direct—such as repaying a debt, or indirect—such as making a commitment to tell the truth in the future. But atonement also has a deeper meaning.

The word "atone" does not come from Hebrew or Latin. Rather, it is an English word that comes from being "at one with" in the sense of "in harmony" or "in accord." It literally means at-one-ment. When our atonement is genuine, we are doing more than acknowledging responsibility for haven caused harm to others. We feel a deep and genuine remorse, because we realize that when we harm others, we also harm ourselves. When we do something wrong, we are driving a wedge between ourselves and others. We are no longer "in harmony" and this causes distress. True atonement can only happen when we are at one with others and with the Higher Power's will for us. Many of us try to make amends for things we have done, without concentrating our efforts on the most important part of atonement—overcoming our isolation. Atonement is a way of overcoming the delusion that we live in a world of our own, apart from the interwoven web of all creation.

Amends and Faith Traditions

Since making amends is essential to spiritual growth, it plays a central role in religious faith. In the *Bible*, God tells the Israelites to atone for their sins, commanding them to set aside one day each year, the tenth day of the seventh month for the Day of Atonement (Leviticus 16:29-30; 23:27-28). On this date, the people were to bring a sin offering, an innocent animal sacrifice "whose blood was brought in to make atonement" (Leviticus 16:27). Today, this day is known as Yom Kippur—the highest of all Jewish holidays. Christians believe that Christ came to earth to atone for the sins of the world, giving up his body and his blood for the salvation of humankind. Christians reenact Christ's sacrifice with the bread and wine of communion. For Catholics, Christ is the very embodiment of atonement—the "Lamb of God who takes away the sins of the world." During the Catholic Mass, priests remind those present that they should not receive communion bread and wine unless they have confessed their sins, and put aside their resentments—especially against those who may have harmed them. The doctrine of atonement is also a central teaching of Islam; there are fourteen verses in the *Koran* on the subject of atonement, and the faithful are commanded to daily prayer, subjugating their own will to that of Allah. Buddhism teaches that true wisdom is found not in the material world around us, but through meditation and contemplation— spiritual practices intended to help followers detach from cravings and resentments which, according to Buddhist doctrine, are the basis of suffering.

In order to move forward with our recovery from chronic pain, we must make an effort to atone for what we have done wrong, or what we failed to do. Whatever our religious beliefs, we must accept the fact that true healing requires a real effort to overcome our negative feelings and move ahead with our lives.

Being Self-Centered

We usually think of individuals as being self-centered if they think only about their needs and not about the needs of others. We call such people selfish and, if they seem to have an overly high opinion of themselves, we may call them conceited. We have all met people who never seem to find any fault with their own actions, but are quick to judge others. Psychologists call such individuals narcissistic, referring to the Greek myth of Narcissus.

According to the myth, Narcissus was rather enamored with himself. The god Nemesis was annoyed with Narcissus and made him look into a pool of water. Seeing his own beautiful reflection in the still water, Narcissus immediately fell in love with the image he saw in the water. Since he had never seen anyone else so beautiful, he continued to stare at his own reflection, growing increasingly miserable and frustrated because he could not be with the one he most loved. Since

Narcissus did not realize that he was looking at his own reflection; he presumed it was someone else. Eventually, he died alone and in love only with himself.

Could it be that we have more in common with Narcissus than we might first think? Most of us would say that we are hardly stuck on ourselves. Quite the contrary, many of us have come to see ourselves as defective, broken, or less worthwhile than others. We cannot possibly be narcissistic, can we? Like Narcissus, we are often alone, cut off from the world around us. We may not be staring at a beautiful reflection in a pond, but we may be constantly thinking about our suffering, avoiding contact with others, and preoccupied mostly with our own concerns. This is a form of narcissism. Oblivious to his surroundings, Narcissus stared at his own reflection in the water. Unless we accept the fact that we have purpose in the world, and this purpose involves connection with others, we may live our lives much as Narcissus did—trapped in mistaken beliefs. We may spend our lives self-absorbed, and die without knowing who we were really meant to be. In order to atone, we must overcome our isolation and become at-one with the world.

Amends to Ourselves—Allowing Ourselves to Laugh

The idea that humor and laughter can help reduce pain is hardly new. What is new is that modern medicine is beginning to seriously consider the healing value of humor. Chronic pain often leads to a preoccupation with our own situation; laughter can help us overcome self-centeredness or the overly serious disposition that so often accompanies chronic pain.

What is humor? Although people sometimes laugh to themselves, they are much more likely to laugh when in the company of others. Laughter is infectious. When one person laughs, others often join in. Scientists do not view laughter as a simple reflex; rather, it is best described as a learned autonomic response. Jokes are funny as long as we don't know the punch line because the stimulus for laughter is the realization that things are not what we expected. In this way, humor helps us see things in a new or different way. We laugh at ourselves when we are surprised at something we did or said—usually when it was a mistake. This kind of humor is a sign of maturity and self-acceptance because we are acknowledging that we goof up from time to time.

There are types of humor that are not healthy. Humor that belittles others often takes the form of sarcastic or ethnic jokes. Laughing at the expense of others is wrong since it reinforces the distorted view that we are better than others. We need to move past negative humor in order to make progress in our recovery.

Keeping our sense of humor alive and well is important to developing a hopeful, positive attitude. Our happiness is greatly influenced by the way we choose to look at misfortune. Rather than focus on the negative, we must try to discover an upside for what seems like a bad situation. The choice is ours. A good laugh relaxes our body and mind and is strong medicine against suffering.

Inspirational Reading—Albert Schweitzer

"As far back as I can remember I was saddened by the amount of misery I saw in the world around me. Youth's unqualified joie de vivre, *I never really knew, and I believe that to be the*

case with many children, even though they appear outwardly merry and quite free from care."

"It was quite incomprehensible to me—this was before I began going to school—why in my evening prayers, I should pray for human beings only. So, when my mother had prayed with me and had kissed me good night, I used to silently add a prayer that I had composed myself for all living creatures. It ran thus: 'O, heavenly Father, protect and bless all things that have breath; guard them from all evil, and let them sleep in peace."

"He comes to us as One unknown, without a name, as of old, by the lake side, He came to those men who knew Him not. He speaks to us the same word: 'Follow thou me!' and sets us to the tasks, which He has to fulfill for our time. He commands. And to those who obey Him, whether they be wise or simple, He will reveal Himself in the toils, the conflicts, the sufferings, which they shall pass through in His fellowship, and, as an ineffable mystery, they shall learn in their own experience Who He is."

Albert Schweitzer was born in the Alsace region that is now part of France. His father was a minister and both of his grandfathers were talented organists. Schweitzer began intensive religious studies at the University of Strasbourg in 1893, and he received a doctorate degree in 1899. He began preaching at St. Nicholas Church in Strasbourg in this same year, and went on to academic positions at the University of Strasbourg, where he achieved recognition as a biblical scholar. Following his father's example, he began a distinguished musical career, composing organ music for religious service. He also wrote a biography of the composer J.S. Bach in both French and German.

Albert Schweitzer could have rested on his laurels and lived the comfortable life of a university professor, but this was not his calling. He decided to leave his academic career to become a medical missionary. In 1905, he entered medical school so he could fulfill this ministry. In 1913, having obtained his medical degree, he founded his hospital at Lambaréné in what was then French Equatorial Africa. To do this, he had to give up the comforts and security of his home and academic appointment, and he had to face criticism from fellow clergy who questioned his religious beliefs. During World War I, both he and his wife were sent to a French internment camp as prisoners of war. Conditions there were quite difficult.

In 1924, Schweitzer returned to Africa, where he would spend the rest of his life. He served as chief doctor, pastor of a congregation, administrator of a village, superintendent of buildings and grounds, writer of scholarly books, and musician for those who lived nearby! In 1952, he received the Nobel Peace Prize. He continued to work until his death in 1965.

Albert Schweitzer was one of the greatest humanitarians of the twentieth century. He endured discomfort, personal risk, professional criticism, and internment in a prison camp in order to live life in accordance with the will of the Higher Power as he understood it. For us, Schweitzer can serve a symbol of triumph of the spirit over the obstacles created by national, cultural, ethnic, and religious differences. Schweitzer recognized that medicine alone was not sufficient to heal the suffering of chronic illness—that true healing required attending to emotional and spiritual well-being of his patients. Thus, even as our bodies age and become weak, we can follow Schweitzer's example and continue to grow in mind and spirit.

Ninth Step Prayer

I pray for the right attitude to make my amends, being mindful not to harm others in the process. I pray for the strength, courage and direction to do the right thing, no matter what the personal consequences may be. I pray not to delay if it can be avoided.

Exercises for the Ninth Step

Humor Exercises

Comedy films– Make a point of seeing at least one comedy movie or show each week. It is best to share this experience with others. Consider watching it with a school-age child, perhaps a grandchild, niece, or nephew. Children are much less critical than are adults, and they enjoy silly, slapstick routines. Notice whether you find yourself sharing in their laughter. Notice whether your pain is less while you were watching the film. How did you feel afterwards?

Making mistakes–We all goof up from time to time. These are usually not serious, life-altering events. For the perfectionists or overly seriously individuals among us, learning to laugh at our own mistakes is good medicine. Is it such a big deal to put three instead of two teaspoons of sugar in our morning coffee, or to forget to take out the trash? We need to learn to laugh at life's little mistakes so that the bigger problems we face will not seem like catastrophes.

Take note of the little mistakes you make during each day and write them down.

For each mistake, write down the consequences of the mistake (e.g. your coffee was too sweet).

Try to laugh at your mistakes. At first, this may seem contrived, but as time goes on, you will find that you are conditioning yourself to recognize mistakes for what they are—little surprises in your life that make you laugh!

119

Physical Activity Exercise

Physical pain limits our ability to exercise. Some of us are extremely limited in what we can do. Others are still very active, but have had to give up playing sports they once enjoyed. Scientific research has proven that physical exercise decreases pain and improves our sense of well-being. Each of us can benefit from an exercise program. Exercise increases our endorphins—natural painkillers. Exercise helps maintain strength and flexibility, prevents osteoporosis and can decrease our risk of falling. Despite knowing these facts, many of us have stopped exercising. If we have neglected our bodies, we need to make amends to ourselves. To become optimistic about our future, we must be concerned about our emotional and our physical health.

There are many healthy forms of exercise. Some of us prefer to join health clubs where we can participate in organized classes such as water aerobics, dance, step, Pilates or yoga. Others prefer competitive sports such as tennis or golf. These kinds of activities increase the amount of time we spend with others—helping us overcome social isolation. There are simple forms of exercise we can do alone such as swimming, walking, biking, gardening, or using home exercise equipment. Any exercise that we enjoy is good exercise, provided we begin gradually and don't overdo it, but checking with a doctor before starting a new program is advisable.

Physical Activity Diary

Some of us have abused our bodies. We may have damaged our lungs by smoking cigarettes, or developed liver damage because of alcohol or drug abuse. We may have overindulged in food or gone on crazy diets. Now is the time to make

120

amends for abusing our bodies. Now we must commit to a healthy diet and to regular exercise.

Over the next few weeks, keep a log of your physical activity. If you are not used to exercising, begin slowly. If you are not sure of your current exercise capacity or cardiovascular health, consult your physician. There is no need for a structured exercise program, such as scheduled gym workouts; just increasing daily physical activity is a good start. Take note of your current activity level and gauge your progress over the next few weeks. As an example, you might choose to walk up stairs instead of using an elevator. Continue to record your daily activity in a journal or chart. You might even consider giving yourself a reward for increasing activity. Of course, this reward should be something healthy. Consider a reward that involves another person, so that you can celebrate your achievement together—perhaps a movie, show, or dinner.

Example:

Day of the Week: Monday

Time of day: 9 a.m.—10 a.m.

Type of activity: Walking

Activity achievement: 2.1 miles

Pain during exercise (0-10): 3/10

Pain after exercise (0-10): 2/10

Mood after exercises (0-10): 8/10

Energy level (0-10): 6/10

Overcoming Unhealthy Thinking Exercise

This exercise helps us overcome negative thinking. In Step 4, we made a list of our strengths and weaknesses. Now we need to review our lists before proceeding with this exercise. Write down your negative beliefs about yourself. One commonly held belief among those with chronic pain is "I am useless." The example below shows how to challenge this mistaken notion. For each negative belief, follow the same format as the example below:

Automatic Thought: I am practically useless as a wife; it's a wonder my husband stays with me.

Negative Belief behind the Automatic Thought: If I cannot shop for groceries, then my husband has to do it and he hates shopping.

Reason for this belief: Shopping for food has always been my responsibility. Because of my neck and shoulder pain, I can't lift grocery bags. I can't do the things a wife should do.

Consider alternative ways of looking at this situation, for example:

-I cannot change the fact that I hurt too much to carry groceries right now, but there are other things I can do to help my family.

-Rather than shopping once a week, I can make more frequent trips to the store and carry small packages.

-Times are changing; maybe it is a good thing that my husband has to adjust to new ways of sharing responsibilities. He might even find that he enjoys shopping.

-Shopping on days when I cook can help me to find the freshest vegetables and best bargains.

Action Steps to Affirm Self-worth

I can discuss division of duties with my husband.

I can spend more time reviewing our son's homework.

I can balance the checkbook.

I can do light housekeeping duties such as dusting and vacuuming.

I can make a shopping list and join my husband when he shops.

I can shop for vegetables and light grocery items during the week.

Repeat this process for each of your negative beliefs. Share this exercise with a friend, sponsor, or therapist.

Chapter 10

Continuing to Take Responsibility

Chronic Pain Step 10: Continue to take personal inventory of our strengths and our weaknesses, and promptly admit when we harm others or ourselves.

Marianne's Story

"I am a 35-year-old woman with chronic neck pain treated with medications and counseling for over a year. I was diagnosed with herniated discs and pinched nerves that caused shooting pains down my arm. I tried injections and other treatments, but my pain continued. At first, I resisted the idea that my emotions were part of the problem. Now I know better.

I am an adult child of an alcoholic father. When I was little, I learned that it was safer to keep my feelings to myself. I also learned to become a caretaker—someone who pays too much attention to others' needs and not enough attention to her own. This often happens in children of alcoholics. When I was a girl, I spent a lot of time worrying about my mother and father. I also had to look after my brothers and sisters.

I have come to realize that I have been too hard on myself. I blame myself for things that went wrong in my family life when there was more than enough blame to go around. I am still hard on myself at times, but I am able to snap out of it. When I find myself worrying, I ask myself what I am feeling. The answer is usually fear; I am afraid that the worst possible thing that can happen will happen. The fear becomes worry, so I rehash things over and over again in my head. Now, I take the time to write down my feelings. I write 'I am afraid.' Then, I write down the reason why I am afraid. I tell myself, "This is only a feeling—I am afraid, but I can get past this fear." Then I consider other possibilities besides the worst-case scenario. I usually find that I am treating life's little problems as big catastrophes. When I consider other outcomes, my fear goes away. Sure, I have bad days, but I am gradually learning to live one day at a time."

Continuing to Monitor our Beliefs, Feelings, and Actions

It is easy to fall into the trap of complacency. We have made progress in our recovery, and having suffered so much for so long, it is tempting to accept things the way they are. Unless we are vigilant in keeping an inventory of our strengths and our weaknesses, we can easily slip back into old patterns of unhealthy thinking and behavior. This is a well-recognized problem in all Twelve Step programs. Some who attend AA figure they have the problem licked after 90 days of sobriety, so they stop going to meetings and relapse within a few weeks. AA teaches that no one is recovered—only recovering. In a similar way, chronic pain is a condition that cannot be cured. Recovery requires regular practice of relaxation, meditation, and positive thinking techniques we have learned. When we become complacent, we risk falling back into our old, unhealthy ways of coping with pain. We might find ourselves losing our spiritual focus, perhaps falling to the temptations of modern day idols—false gods.

False Gods

The *Bible* story of Exodus retells the trials and tribulations of the Jewish people in their Egyptian captivity and their exodus across the Red Sea into the Sinai. The Jewish people had suffered greatly in Egypt. They suffered physical pain as they toiled under the yoke of slavery, and they suffered the emotional pain from loss of their homeland and their freedom. It was not only the Jewish people who suffered. Exodus tells us that God sent many plagues upon the Egyptian people. With crops lost to locusts, they suffered hunger. With bodies ravaged by boils, they suffered pain. Worse still, they suffered the anguish of losing their first-born sons. Finally, the Egyptian Pharaoh relented and allowed the Jewish people to return to their homeland.

After all of their trials and tribulations, one would expect that the newly freed Jewish people would be resolute in their faithfulness to God, but this was hardly the case. Moses went up Mount Sinai to receive the Ten Commandments—a covenant or agreement between God and his people written on two stone tablets by the hand of God, but upon his return from the mountain, Moses found his people worshiping a false idol—a golden calf. In anger, Moses threw down the tablets, shattering them into many pieces. God sent a plague upon the people as punishment for their wrongdoing. After repentance, God is reconciled with his people and again writes the covenant on two new stone tablets. The Israelites built the Arc of the Covenant to hold the broken pieces of the original stone tablets as well as the two new tablets. They then carried the Arc on their journey to Palestine as a reminder of their obligations and that God is with them.

This story of the Exodus has meaning for us today as it did for the Jewish people over 2,500 years ago. We no longer worship golden calves, but we do worship false gods. We lose conscious contact with the Higher Power when we are distracted by modern day idols. We think success or wealth will make us happy, whole, and fulfilled. We believe we can find real meaning in new clothes, new cars, bigger televisions, new lovers, or the success of our favorite sports teams. There is nothing wrong with any of these things, just as there is nothing wrong with statues of calves. What is wrong is the worship of these things. In these twelve steps, we honestly admit our shortcomings and pledge to correct them. Like the Israelites, we turn to the Higher Power for guidance.

As individuals, we are in need of emotional and spiritual healing, but our society is also in need of healing. As we stop worshiping false gods and learn to heed the Higher Power, the world becomes a better place for all of humankind. As we heal our emotional and spiritual wounds, we become healthier, and, at the same time, we also help heal society. We must learn to accept that chronic physical pain is a part of our lives that we cannot control, but also to accept that our pain has brought to our attention the need to renew our covenant with the Higher Power.

Developing Healthy Relationships

Recovery is based on self-awareness, honesty, trust, and openness. Relationships are important measures of our progress. We may need to monitor how we interact with others—especially family, friends, and coworkers. We have learned that chronic pain can interfere with our relationships. Relationships are like plants in a vegetable garden; if we neglected our garden, we will soon discover that weeds have taken over. Like gardeners, we must cultivate our relationships, look for signs of distress, and tend to any problems that arise. As we monitor our progress, we shall be always vigilant for signs of complacency.

Healthy relationships do not come easily for many of us. In Twelve Step programs, newcomers are cautioned not to form any new romantic relationships until they are secure in recovery—usually a year of sobriety for those who are addicted to drugs or alcohol. Romantic relationships can be particularly difficult and confusing because they present us with romantic attachment, sex drives and dependency issues. When recovering from chronic pain, it is best to use caution in forming new romantic relationships until we are "solid" in our pain management program.

Inspirational Readings—Viktor Emil Frankl

"The salvation of man is through love and in love. I understood how a man who has nothing left in this world still may know bliss, be it only for a brief moment, in the contemplation of his beloved."

"What man actually needs is not a tensionless state, but rather the striving and struggling for some goal worthy of him. What he needs is not the discharge of tension at any cost, but the call of a potential meaning waiting to be fulfilled by him."

Viktor Frankl was born in Vienna, Austria. When he was in high school, he became very interested in the workings of the mind and began corresponding with Sigmund Freud—the father of psychiatry. Freud recognized young Frankl's abilities. Following in Freud's footsteps, Frankl attended medical school in Vienna, graduating in 1925.

Early in his career, Frankl began developing his own theories about personality and emotional illness. In 1928, Frankl organized cost-free counseling centers for teenagers in Vienna and six other cities. In 1933, he was charged with supervising a psychiatric unit for suicidal women. In 1937, Frankl opened a private psychiatric practice. One year later, Hitler's troops invaded Austria and his life was forever changed. For a while, he worked at the only hospital for Jews in Vienna. When the Nazis began killing mentally ill patients as "undesirables," Frankl falsified medical records to keep his patients from being executed.

In 1942, the Nazi's arrested Frankl and his young wife, taking them to a concentration camp. He would spend three years as prisoner number 119-104. Dr. Victor Frankl had gone from being a well-known Vienna psychiatrist to a number in the Nazi's slave labor and genocide machine.

How did Victor Frankl survive? One thing is clear—he did not give up hope. Knowing that he would be unable to take any possessions with him, he decided to sew a manuscript into the lining of his coat. That manuscript represented his life's work and he had hoped to soon publish, but he was forced to discard the coat when the Nazi's took him to the Auschwitz concentration camp. What could he do?

Victor Frankly did not give up hope, as so many others did. While in Auschwitz, he tried to find a way to continue his work against all odds. Frankl began to reconstruct his manuscript in his head, and then wrote what he could on scraps of paper that he found. Separated from his wife and family, and not knowing whether they were alive or dead, Frankl could have given up his will to live. He realized that his family members were still with him in spirit, though not in body. He used the knowledge of their love for each other to sustain him during his long, terrible ordeal. In observing other prisoners, Frankl realized that it was those like him—those who held onto a vision of a future—who were most likely to survive in the concentration camp. Frankl came to understand that there is meaning in all of life, even in pain and suffering. It was the fact that prisoners could find meaning under the most terrible, degrading conditions that most impressed him. Suffering was part of their experience.

There are many things in life that we are powerless to change, but for Dr. Frankl and other concentration camp prisoners, there was next to nothing they could change. Even the Nazis could not strip away Frankl's humanity. He maintained hope and moral behavior in the face of hopelessness and immorality. He concluded that it is our very approach toward life's adversity that makes us truly human. After the concentration camps were liberated, Frankl soon learned that his loved ones had all perished. In spite of his grief, he resumed medical practice in Vienna, and continued his research and writing. His book, *Man's Search for Meaning* has sold over nine million copies. Though Victor Frankl is no longer living, his life and work remain an inspiration to others who face terrible adversity in their own lives.

Prayer for the Tenth Step

I pray that I may continue to grow in understanding and effectiveness; To take daily inventories of myself, to correct mistakes when I make them, to take responsibility for my actions, to be ever aware of my negative and self-defeating attitudes and behaviors, to keep my willfulness in check, to keep love and tolerance of others as my code and to continue in daily prayer.

Exercise for the Tenth Step

In order to assess your current relationships, answer each of the following questions:

-Do you isolate from people who care for you?

-Do you criticize people who are important in your life?

-Are you distrustful of loved ones?

-Do you spend too much time worrying about what someone thinks about you?

-Are you afraid to "be yourself" when around others?

-Does your mind race so fast that you are not aware of what is going on around you??

-Are you able to honestly tell others what you need from them?

-When you make a mistake, do you promptly admit it?

-Do you often complain about your situation?

-Do you dwell on your limitations rather than your abilities??

If the answer to any of these questions is "yes", what can you do about it?

Chapter 11

Becoming Aware of Purpose in Our Lives

Chronic Pain Step 11: Sought through prayer and meditation to improve our conscious contact with our Higher Power, praying only for knowledge of our Higher Power's will for us and for the power to carry that out.

Stephen's Story

"Although I still have neck pain, and I may need to have an operation, I am no longer suffering. Two years ago, I considered myself disabled. That was before I entered a comprehensive pain program where I learned to manage my pain. Now I accept the fact that I have a bad neck, and I always will. I am also resigned to the fact that I will never return to my old job. However, I am not going to die from arthritis in my neck. I have my life to live. I have a wonderful, loving family—the center of my life. I have learned to take life a little less seriously, to appreciate what I have, and to let go of my anger. I have learned to pray and to turn my problems over to my Higher Power.

Last week, I had to go before a judge about my disability. Before I was treated in the pain program, I would have let this eat me up. I would have been frightened and angry. My neck muscles would have gone into spasm just thinking about it. But now it is different. I feel good about how much I've accomplished. I have learned to manage my pain with medication, exercises, relaxation, distraction, affirmations, and other techniques I learned in the pain program."

Becoming Aware of the Purpose in Our Lives

The Eleventh Step requires us to pray or meditate in order to improve our conscious contact with the Higher Power. Despite having progressed through the preceding Steps, some of us still question how spiritual practice can help overcome suffering. When we pray or meditate, we elevate our level of thinking beyond ourselves—overcoming the illusion that we are alone in the world. The more we dwell on ourselves, the more we trap ourselves in the prison of our own making. Trying to "go it alone" doesn't work. Self-reliance is an illusion that makes us arrogant, angry, stubborn, and miserable. Prayer—going to the Higher Power—frees us from the bondage of our worries and fears. Meditation—increasing our conscious awareness—frees us from constant worry and unhealthy attachment. Spiritual growth occurs slowly and through discipline. We learn to rely on the Higher Power for guidance. Over time, we become more confident that the Higher Power is with us.

From time to time, we may face problems that seem overwhelming. We may find ourselves slipping into resentment, anger, self-pity, or worry. This is when we most need to pray. In prayer, we ask the Higher Power to help us overcome our negative feelings and to show us the way. At such times, we might also meditate, read spiritual writings, do charity work or just stop and rest. If we find ourselves unable to let go of our problem, we ask the Higher Power for strength to help us get through the difficult times. As we continue to pray, we will see that our old way of living becomes more outdated and unattractive. Problems do not seem as difficult as they once did. We begin to find new ways of living. We become more spontaneous. Life becomes easier and we begin to experience real peace.

Some of us find that prayer comes quite naturally, while others are completely put off by the idea of praying. Many of our attitudes and beliefs about prayer were formed during childhood. We may have memorized prayers before we understood their meaning. We may have recited The Lord's Prayer before we could read, hardly understanding the meaning of such words as "hallowed" or "trespass." Prayers such as, "Now I lay me down to sleep," may have been frightening to us children, especially the line: "If I die before I wake, I pray the Lord my soul to take." As children, some of us were encouraged to pray for material things—a new bicycle for example. If we did get a new bicycle, it probably was not a direct result of prayer. We may have prayed in school for a candidate to win an election, and now, as adults, this seems more like manipulation. Some of us may have prayed for God to make our parents stop fighting, and, when our prayers were not answered, may have lost faith or even became angry with God. If we are not comfortable with prayer, it is time to reevaluate why.

Those of us who are sports fans are used to seeing teams gather around the coach or chaplain and pray before a sports contest. Pre-game prayers by the St. Bartholomew High School basketball team are not likely to decide the winner. If they are not praying for divine intervention in the game's outcome, then why pray at all? Can prayer actually help basketball players and the team play better? Of course, they can. Why? Because prayer helps us change what we believe, how we feel, and how we act. Consider the basketball player's prayers below:

> "God, I am afraid before each basketball game. I know that I do not play well when I am too nervous. I know that I am afraid of messing up and of what people might think. Please help me overcome my fears. Help me understand that it is okay to make mistakes, and that I am no less in your eyes for having done so, as long as I've tried my best."

> "God, I need help with my anger. During last week's game, I shoved another player and was kicked out of the game. I need to control my anger. Please help me remain calm, and help me stay cool when another player tries to provoke me."

> "God, I need your help in facing defeat. I know that basketball is just a game, and that we cannot always win. But I get bummed out for days after we lose. I get so moody that I sometimes snap at my parents for no good reason."

> "God, I need your help with organizing my time. I should get my homework done in study hall, and then I would have more time to practice my shooting drills in the gym. I have never been good at sticking to plans. I could use some help with this."

Coaches certainly understand the power of positive thinking. And coaches in religious schools will make use of the power of prayer as a positive force in young adults' lives. High school basketball players with religious faith can use prayer to increase their conscious contact with the Higher Power. They may be asking for help with beliefs (e.g. It is okay to make a mistake.), feelings (fear and anger), and actions (shoving other players, planning study time). Whether one believes in the concept of a God, Spirit, Consciousness, Creation, Higher Self or any other concept of a Higher Power, spiritual practice is important to our recovery.

Quieting the Busy Mind

It is almost impossible to connect with the Higher Power if we are constantly in a state of hyper-drive. Racing thoughts distract us from work, our relationships with others, and our relationship with the Higher Power. Sometimes racing thoughts keep us awake at night, so we are tired and worn out during the day. This just adds to our fatigue and our pain. Mind racing deceives us into thinking that we are in control because we are busy thinking about problems, but rarely changes anything.

For some of us, regular exercise or meditation is effective in slowing down the hyperactive brain. For others, our minds are racing so fast that we are not able to slow down enough to sit still for meditation, and we continue to mind race even while exercising. Those of us with mind racing that does not improve with meditation or exercise should consult a physician. Mind racing may be a sign of a medical problem such as bipolar (manic-depressive) illness—a condition requiring mood-stabilizing medication. Often, mind racing comes from childhood emotional injury. When we were children, we may have experienced unpleasant or traumatic events. Children have little power, especially over adults, so they turn to their imagination. Using their imagination, children replay versions of unpleasant events repeatedly in their minds to make things seem okay. By thinking about these events, children try convincing themselves they were not to blame, or that the painful event did not happen the way they remembered, or that they would be more prepared to deal with it better next time. Mind racing is one way children cope. Unlike children, adults *do* have power—often more than they realize—and the mind racing habit of childhood is no longer productive. Mind racing gives us the illusion of control, and it keeps us so busy that we do not have to deal with our feelings. It robs us of our strength. Meditation helps us overcome mind racing and create space for the Higher Power in our lives.

Inspirational Reading- Wilma Rudolph

"I tell them that the most important aspect is to be yourself and have confidence in yourself... I remind them that triumph can't be had without the struggle."

Wilma Rudolph was an African-American born in rural Tennessee—the 20th of 22 children! Her father was a railway porter, and her mother did housework for wealthy white families. Her family was very poor, but her parents did what they could to provide for their children. What they could not provide in material goods, they more than made up for with love, hope, encouragement, and faith.

As a young child, Wilma was stricken with polio—a disease that causes paralysis. During her rehabilitation, Wilma was fitted with a metal leg brace so that she could walk. When Wilma attended grade school, Tennessee was still segregated, so African-American and white students attended separate schools. Wilma attended to her studies and participated in physical recreation activities, especially with her athletically-gifted older sisters. With the encouragement of family and friends, Wilma strengthened her leg. By age 12, she was able to walk without crutches, braces, or corrective shoes.

Wilma Rudolph wanted to participate in team sports like her older sisters. She did not let braces and crutches stop her from pursuing her dream. When she gave up her leg brace, she joined a local basketball team, but did not play in a single game for next three years. Wilma continued to become stronger as she grew. By the time she was in high school, she had become a basketball star, setting state records for scoring and leading her team to a state championship. Wilma knew she could run fast, but her high school did not have money to support a track team. The coach of the famous Tennessee State University Tigerbells track team noticed how fast she was when he came to see a basketball game. He invited Wilma to a sports camp the following summer, and she was given a scholarship to Tennessee State where she became an immediate star. In 1960, Wilma attended Olympic trials and she set a world record in the 200-meter run that stood for eight years. In Rome, she became the first American woman to win three gold medals in the Olympic Games. She won the 100-meter dash, the 200-meter dash, and she ran anchor on the winning 400-meter relay team. When she returned home, Wilma was greeted by her team and a parade in her honor— the first integrated event in the city's history.

Wilma Rudolph went on to become a schoolteacher and a track coach. She also became an inspiration to men and women all over the world as someone who had overcome polio, poverty, and discrimination to become one of the most recognized and admired individuals of her generation.

Eleventh Step Prayer

I pray for help me in freeing my mind of distracting worries and concerns. I pray for help in overcoming anger, resentment, self-pity, and self-centeredness. I pray for guidance in my decision-making and to be free of the bondage of willfulness.

Exercises for the Eleventh Step

Prayer Exercise I

There are many ways to pray. Some pray as part of a religious service. If you attend a religious service or a Twelve Step group that closes with a prayer, notice how you feel immediately afterwards. Do you feel you are closer to your Higher Power? Do you feel more at peace? Are you less aware of your pain?

Make a list of your prayers. How are these prayers important to your recovery from suffering? How do you feel when you are praying to your Higher Power for help?

In Twelve Step meetings, we often hear people say that they have turned over their lives to a Higher Power, trusting that things will work out. They know that prayers are not answered immediately. Sometimes, solutions to problems just seem to appear as if out of nowhere. How does the Higher Power answer your prayers?

From time to time, we all become discouraged and lose hope. This is when we most need to pray. Have you developed a routine that helps maintain your connection with your Higher Power? Are you sometimes angry with your Higher Power? If so, how do you deal with this anger?

Through working the Twelve Step program, we become grateful for the gifts of life. How do you express gratitude?

Prayer Exercise II

Review your inventory of strengths and weaknesses. For each item on your list, write a prayer or positive affirmative on an index card. Keep these index cards with you at all times, and commit to reading them at least four times a day. As you do this, you will be increasing your conscious connection with the Higher Power. Do not expect miracles. It took a long time to develop negative beliefs and feelings; they will not disappear overnight. But the more you affirm the positive, the easier it will become. Try it! What have you got to lose?

Examples:

Helplessness—I will find the courage to try new ways of getting my needs met.

Resentment—Higher Power, help me overcome my anger and resentments. Yours is the way of love and forgiveness, not of anger and reprisal.

Self-Pity—I accept the fact that I have pain, and help me find the strength to put my suffering in proper perspective and overcome self-pity.

Attention-Seeking—Higher Power, I have used my illness as a way to get attention from others. Help me learn to express my needs in a genuine way, and not manipulate others.

Perfectionism—Higher Power, help me accept the fact that to err is indeed human. No one can be perfect, and holding unattainable standards just gives me an excuse to criticize myself, or others for failing to reach them.

Fear of Failure—Higher Power, I use my illness as an excuse for not trying. I am afraid of failing. Help me overcome my fears, so that I might carry out your will for me.

Blame—Higher Power, help me accept responsibility for my actions, and not seek comfort by blaming others. I can only be true to your will when I accept responsibility for what I say or do.

Mind Racing Exercise

If you find yourself mind racing, say the simple prayer "Higher Power, help me stop mind racing." There are legitimate concerns that need to be addressed, but mind racing is a waste of time. Set aside a specific time of the day for legitimate problem solving. In the coming weeks, say this prayer often, especially when your mind turns to negative thoughts. Remind yourself that you have a time and place for planning and problem solving. This simple technique is useful any time you are dealing with intrusive, repetitive, and nonproductive thoughts.

Worry Journal

Begin keeping a worry journal. Keep it with you throughout the day. Describe your worries in detail. Although journaling will not fix problems, it may make them seem more manageable. The mere act of writing down concerns may create a safety zone between you and your thoughts so you will be less controlled by them. You may also learn that many of your worries are exaggerated.

Chapter 12

Helping Others Overcome Suffering

Chronic Pain Step 12: Having had a spiritual awakening as a result of these steps, we sought to carry this message to others and to practice these principles in all of our affairs.

Suzanne's Story

"I can hardly believe how my life has changed. I was a 40-year-old woman with uncontrolled chronic pain resorted to buying pills from friends and acquaintances. Now I have come to understand that I was using pain pills to dull my physical pain as well as my emotional pain. I was hooked. Now I have my life back.

I have learned to recognize my fear and call it what it is— just a feeling. If fear doesn't pass, I pick up the phone and call a friend or I talk with my husband. If I feel sad, I call it what it is—just a feeling. If the sadness doesn't pass, I tell myself that out of sadness comes strength and understanding. I have learned that everything happens for a reason, even bad things. I have learned to trust in my Higher Power.

When I was young, I was sexually molested. For a long time, I believed that the abuse had ruined my life. Now I know that my pain and suffering have given me insight and compassion. I volunteer to help other women who were sexually abused. I help them grow in mind and spirit, and to live one day at a time. The Twelve-Steps have given me back my life. Now I understand God's will for me."

Helping Others Overcome Suffering

When we began our twelve step journey, we found ourselves trapped in a prison of our own making—a prison where the cell door bars were made of bitterness, resentment, hopelessness, distrust, and fear. With the help of the Higher Power, we are now free from our prison. Having had a spiritual awakening, we now help others set themselves free. By helping others overcome suffering, we make the world a better place for all. This is not an option; it is a natural result of letting the Higher Power work within us.

In school, we learned about famous kings, queens, prime ministers and presidents who took bold steps to make their countries better. It is natural to assume they were important people but we are not. This is an illusion. Political leaders reflect the beliefs and opinions of the society in which they live. As society changes through the efforts of individuals like us, political leaders change their viewpoints. In overcoming our own fears and making room for the Higher Power in our lives, we make the world a better place.

The American civil rights leader Rev. Martin Luther King, Jr. understood the power of transforming suffering and oppression into a force for change. Those of us old enough to remember the Civil Rights Movement of the 1960's are struck by how much the United States has changed in the last half century. Before the civil rights movement, much of the country denied African-Americans access to restaurants, theaters, public swimming pools, and state universities. Rev. King preached the principles of nonviolence developed by Mahatma Gandhi. He brought attention to the injustice of the time, and to the courage of those who practiced nonviolence. Both Gandhi and Rev. King organized the poor and oppressed against the state by asserting human rights over unjust laws. Both leaders were imprisoned. Both accepted that in their pursuit of justice they risked death, and both were killed by an assassin's bullet. Gandhi once said, "Fear is not a disease of the body; fear kills the soul."

The notion that the oppressed, poor, and infirm have a special role to play in society is hardly new. Christian and non-Christian scholars agree that this is a central theme in the Gospels of the *New Testament*. At the time of Christ, Judea (modern Israel) was ruled by the puppet government of Herod, propped up by the Roman Empire. The empire was built upon a foundation of conquest, slave labor, rule by force and fear. It would have been very difficult for anyone to convince Herod or Caesar to reform the Roman Empire. Though historians and religious scholars hold differing beliefs about the divinity of Christ, they agree that he was a reformer. Christ's program was not aimed at the overthrow of a dictatorship through force or coercion.

Christ ministered directly to the oppressed, poor, and infirm. He taught that those poor in spirit—not the proud—would inherit the kingdom of God, as opposed to the kingdom (Empire) of Caesar. Christ taught that: "The first shall be last and the last shall be first." He taught that it was harder for the rich to enter the kingdom of God than for the poor. How could this be so?

Christians regard Christ as the Messiah or anointed one. The oppressed Jewish people had been waiting for just such a person. Some thought that the Messiah would be a warrior king, who like King David would lead the Jewish people in revolt against the Romans. Others believed that the coming of the Messiah marked the end of time. Christ was not a warrior king, but he was a revolutionary. He challenged the political and religious order of the day through his teaching and his ministry. He ignored the prevailing beliefs about class distinction by ministering to the Jewish equivalents of untouchables—lepers, toll collectors, and prostitutes. He ignored Temple rules that supported the prevailing class structure, violating dietary rules and dining with social outcasts. Christ overturned the tables of the moneylenders in order to make the Temple accessible for worship to all—including those who could not afford to sacrifice at its altar. Clearly, Christ represented a threat to the ruling class who thought that killing him would end their problem. Christians believe that Christ chose to sacrifice himself for the sins of the world, rising from the dead as proof of his divinity and of his teachings.

All societies are in need of reform. The Higher Power works through the lives of each of us, but those who suffer have a special role in transforming society. With war, misfortune, and injustice in the daily news, we often lose perspective. It seems as though things are getting worse. This is not the case. It most industrialized countries it is no longer okay to have segregated schools, pay women a lower wage than men for the same job, or to build public facilities that cannot accommodate those with disabilities. Did all of this change because of the efforts of a few leaders? No. This changed because a few leaders were influenced by the opinion of the many who had already come to know that such inequality was morally wrong. As we open our hearts to love and overcome our fears, we begin to see the world more clearly. We begin to see right and wrong, good and evil more clearly, and can differentiate between the two. We gain the courage to stand up for what is right. We find our voice, as Rev. King and Gandhi found theirs, when we allow the Higher

Power to work through us. We each must do our part in making this world a better place. Leaders will emerge among us, but they cannot succeed without our strength and hope.

Inspirational Readings—Mother Theresa

"There is much suffering in the world– physical, material, mental. The suffering of some can be blamed on the greed of others. The material and physical suffering is suffering from hunger, from homelessness, from all kinds of diseases. But the greatest suffering is being lonely, feeling unloved, having no one. I have come more and more to realize that it is being unwanted that is the worst disease that any human being can ever experience."

"Spread love everywhere you go: first of all in your own house. Give love to your children, to your wife or husband, to a next-door neighbor. . . Let no one ever come to you without leaving better and happier. Be the living expression of God's kindness; kindness in your face, kindness in your eyes, kindness in your smile, kindness in your warm greeting."

"It is not how much we do, but how much love we put in the doing. It is not how much we give, but how much love we put in the giving."

Mother Theresa was born August 27, 1910, in Macedonia as Agnes Gonxha Bojaxhiu. Her father was a contractor, and her mother a homemaker. Her family had a deep religious faith, and was generous to the poor and disadvantaged. By the age of 12, Mother Theresa had decided that her vocation was caring for the poor. At age 18, she joined the Sisters of Loretto order in Ireland; one year later, she went to a convent in India. Mother Theresa spent the next 17 years teaching high school in India.

In 1946, Mother Theresa's life changed forever. She was suspected of having tuberculosis. At that time, there were no antibiotics to treat the disease, but doctors believed that the thin mountain air was one effective treatment. While riding a train to the mountain town of Darjeeling, she received a call from God to serve the poorest of the poor and received permission from the Catholic Church to leave her religious order and move to Calcutta's slums where she set up a school for the poor.

Mother Theresa went on to found the Missionaries of Charity, an order devoted to caring for the poor, the sick, and the dying. She chose to wear a simple white sari with a blue border, similar to the clothes worn by India's poor. She went on to establish schools, soup kitchens, clinics, orphanages, and hospices. She dedicated every day of her adult life to caring for the sick, dying, crippled, mentally ill, and the unwanted.

Mother Theresa suffered from a number of medical problems, including malaria, tuberculosis, and arthritis before dying of heart disease in 1997. In her lifetime, she was awarded the Nobel Peace Prize and many honorary degrees. She traveled throughout the world, meeting with Chiefs of State and other dignitaries to raise social awareness about the plight of the poor and unwanted. Today, about 4,000 Missionaries of Charity continue Mother Theresa's work all over the world.

Twelfth Step Prayer

I have learned to overcome my suffering. My spiritual growth continues to unfold. I pray that I may be able to give hope to others who suffer from chronic pain. For this opportunity I am grateful. I pray for the strength and wisdom to practice the twelve step principles in all that I do and say, so I can continue to grow in spirit and help others.

Exercise for the Twelfth Step

Actions speak louder than words. The Twelve Steps are a part of action-based program. In order to overcome our suffering, we worked at changing our beliefs, attitudes, and behaviors. We made an inventory of our strengths and weaknesses, shared our inventory with others, prayed for the Higher Power's guidance, and changed the way we lived. We are grateful for the progress we have made in our recovery, and we now take the time to make a list of ways we can spread the message to others.

-Describe a recent situation where you helped another person understand the difference between chronic physical pain and emotional suffering.

-Describe a recent situation where you were able to share the facts of your life with another person.

-How has helping others affected your own physical pain?

-Does helping others keep you from becoming complacent and falling back into bad habits? If so, how?

-Do you feel a stronger connection with the Higher Power when you carry the message to others?

Author's Concluding Remarks

It has been my sincere pleasure to serve as your guide in your quest to achieve peace and healing. It is my hope that you will take the information I have provided and use it to help you in your recovery from suffering and to assist others who struggle with chronic pain.

Remember: There is hope; there is help; there is a better way of living your life—one that can be full of joy, despite the presence of physical pain. All that is required is your willingness to begin the journey of recovery.

End Notes

1. National Council on Compensation Insurance. (February 6, 2004). OxyContin prescribing patterns in workers compensation.

2. Rizzo, J.A. (1998). The labor productivity effects of chronic backache in the United States. Medical Care. 36: 1471-1488

3. Wadell G. Keynote address for the primary care forum. (1996). Low back pain: a twentieth century health care enigma. Spine. 21: 2820-2825.

4. Nelemans, PJ. (2003). Injection therapy for subacute and chronic benign low back pain. Cochrane Database of Systematic Reviews. 3.

5. Merrill D.G. (2003). Hoffman's glasses: evidence-based medicine and the search for quality in the literature of interventional pain management. Reg Anesth Pain Med Regional Anesthesia and Pain Management. 28: 547-560.

6. Weinstein, S.M. (2003). Lumbar epidural injections. The Spine Journal. 3:378-448

7. Cluff, R., et al. (2003). The technical aspects of epidural steroid injections: a national survey. Anesth Analg. 96: 907-908.

8. Goldenberg, D.L., Burckhardt, C., Crofford, L. (2004). Management of the fibromyalgia syndrome. JAMA. 292 (19): 2388-95.

9. Chou, R, Clark, E., Helfand, M. (2003). Comparative efficacy and safety of long-acting opioids for chronic non-cancer pain: a systemic review. J Pain Symptom Manage. 26:1026¬46.

10. Sator-Katzenschlager, S.M,.et al (2003). Does pain relief improve pain behavior and mood in chronic pain patients? Anesh Analg. 97: 791-7.

11. Jensen, M.D., et al. (1994). Magnetic imaging of the lumbar spine in patients without back pain. NEJM. 331: 69-73.

12. Oishi, Y., et al. (2003). Lack of association between lumbar degeneration and osteophyte formation in elderly Japanese women with back pain. Bone. 32: 405-11.

13. O'Connell, M.J., Ryan, M., Powell, T., Eustace, S. (2003). The value of routine MR myelography at MRI of the lumbar spine. Acta Radiol. 44: 665-72.

14. Rollins, G. (2003). Rapid MRI no better than X-ray in the treatment of low back pain. Report on Medical Guidelines & Outcomes Research. 14: 6-7.

15. Videman, T. (2003) No clinical advantage of rapid MRI over radiographs for people with low back pain. Evidence-based Heatlthcare. 7: 198-9.

16. Jarvik, J.G., et al. (2003). Rapid magnetic resonance imaging vs. radiographs for patients with low back pain: a randomized controlled trial. JAMA. 289: 2810-8.

17. Videman, T., Battie, M.C., Gibbons, L.E., Maravilla, K., Manninen, H., Kaprio, J. (2003). Associations between back pain history and lumbar MRI findings. Spine. 28:582-8.

18. Dersh, J., Gatchel, R.J., Polatin, P., Mayer, T. (2002). Prevalence of psychiatric disorders in patients with chronic work-related musculoskeletal pain disability. J Occupational and Environmental Medicine. 44: 459-68

19. Dersh, J. (2002). Chronic pain and psychopathology: research findings and theoretical considerations. Psychosom Med. 64: 773-86.

20. Reich, J., Tupin, J. P. & Abramowitz, S.I. Psychiatric diagnosis of chronic pain patients. Am J Psychiatry. 1983; 140: 1495-1498.

21. Fishbain, D.A., Goldberg, M., Meagher, R., Steele, R., Rosomoff, H. (1986). Male and female chronic pain patients categorized by DSM-III psychiatric diagnostic criteria. Pain. 26: 181-197.

22. Holzberg, A D., Robinson, M.E., Geisser M.E. Gremillion HA. (1996). The effects of depression and chronic pain on psychosocial and physical functioning. Clinical Journal of Pain. 12: 118-124.

23. Lin, E.H., et al. (2003). IMPACT Investigators. Effect of improving depression care on pain and functional outcomes among older adults with arthritis: a randomized controlled trial. JAMA. 290:2428-9.

24. Ong, K.S. & Keng, S.B. (2003). The biological, social, and psychological relationship between depression and chronic pain. Cranio. 21:286-94.

25. Bair, M.J., Robinson, R.L., Katon, W., Kroenke, K. (2003). Depression and pain comorbidity: a literature review. Arch. Intern. Med. Archives of Internal Medicine. 163: 2433-45.

26. Birket-Smith, M. (2001). Somatization and chronic pain. Acta Anaesthesiol Scand. 45: 1114-1120.

27. Breckenridge, J., Clark, J.D. (2003). Patient characteristics associated with opioid versus nonsteroidal anti-inflammatory drug management of chronic low back pain. J Pain. 4: 344-50.

28. Friederich, M.A. (1976). Psychological aspects of chronic pelvic pain. Clinical Obstetrics & Gynecology. 19:399-406.

29. Rosenthal, RH. (1993). Psychology of chronic pelvic pain. Obstet Gynecol Clin North Am. 20:627-42.

30. Bailey, B.E., Freedenfeld, R.N., Kiser, R.S., Gatchel, R.J. (2003). Lifetime physical and sexual abuse in chronic pain patients: psychosocial correlates and treatment outcomes. Disabil Rehabil 25: 331-42, 2003

31. Finestone, H.M. (2001). Chronic pain and healthcare utilization in women with a history of sexual abuse. Child Abuse Negl. 24: 1133.

32. Goldberg, R.T., Pachas, W.N., Keith, D. (1999). Relationship between traumatic events in childhood and chronic pain. Disabil Rehabil. 21:23-30.

33. Goldberg, R.T., Goldstein, R. (2000). A comparison of chronic pain patients and controls on traumatic events in childhood. Disabil Rehabil. 22:756-63.

34. Lampe, A., et al. (2003). Chronic pain syndromes and their relation to childhood abuse and stressful life events. J of Psychosom Res. 54:361-7.

35. Dersh, J., Gatchel, R.J., Polatin, P., Mayer, T. (2002). Prevalence of psychiatric disorders in patients with chronic work-related musculoskeletal pain disability. J Occup Environ Med. 44:459-68.

36.Substance Abuse and Mental Health Services Administration. Results from the 2010 National Survey on Drug Use and Health: volume 1: summary of national findings. Rockville, MD: Substance Abuse and Mental Health Services Administration, Office of Applied Studies; 2011

37. Rosenblum, A., Joseph, H., Fong, C., Kipnis, S., Cleland, C, Portenoy, R.K. (2003). Prevalence and characteristics of chronic pain among chemically dependent patients in methadone maintenance and residential treatment facilities. JAMA. 289(18): 2370-8.

38. Jamison, R.N. (2002). Characteristics of methadone maintenance patients with chronic pain. J Pain Symptom Manage. 19:53-62.

39. Arena, J.G. (2002). Chronic pain: psychological approaches for the front-line clinician. J Clin Psychol. 58:1385-96.

40. Tumlin, T.R. (2001). Treating chronic-pain patients in psychotherapy. J Clin Psychol. 57:1277-88.

41. Nelemans, P.J. (2003). Injection therapy for subacute and chronic benign low back pain. Cochrane Database of Systematic Reviews. 3.

42. Van Tudler, M.W., Ostelo, R.W.J.G., Vlaeyen, J.S.W, Linton, S.J, Morley, S.J, & Assendelft, W.J.J. (2004). Behavioural treatment for chronic low back pain. Cochrane Library of Systemic Reviews. (1).

43. Thieme, K., Gromnica-Ihle, E. & Flor, H. (2003). Operant behavioral treatment of fibromyalgia: a controlled study. Arthritis & Rheumatism. 49:314-20.

44. Goldenberg, D.L., Burckhardt, C., & Crofford, L. (2004). Management of the fibromyalgia syndrome. JAMA. 292 (19): 2388-95.

45. Ouimette, P., Crosby, F., Finney, J.W. & Moos, R.H. (1997). Twelve-step and cognitive-behavioral treatment for substance abuse: A comparison of treatment effectiveness. J Consult Clin Psychol. 65: 230-240.

46. Ouimette, P., Humphreys, K., Moos, R.H., Finney J.W., Cronkite, R & Federman, B. (2001). Self-help group participation among substance use disorder patients with posttraumatic stress disorder. J Subst Abuse Treat. 20: 25-32.

47. Humphreys, K., Moos, R. (2001). Can encouraging substance abuse patients to participate in self-help groups reduce demand for health care? A quasi-experimental study. Alcohol Clin Exp Res. 25: 711-716.

Bibliography

Arberry, (translator) A.J. (1997). The Essential Rumi. Book Sales.

Colameco S, Coren JS, Ciervo, CA. Continuous opioid treatment for chronic noncancer pain: a time for moderation in prescribing. Postgrad Med. 2009;121(4):61-66.

Colameco S, Coren JS. Opioid-induced endocrinopathy. J Am Osteopath Assoc. 2009; 109:20-25

Egan, Eileen. (1994). Suffering into Joy: What Mother Theresa Teaches About True Joy. Servant Pubs (ed.).

Fabry (translator), Joseph. (2000). Viktor Frankl Recollections: An Autobiography. Persius Book Club.

Frankl, Viktor E. (1997). Man's Search for Meaning. Pocket Books.

Gandhi, Mahatma. (1996). The Words of Gandhi. W.W. Norton & Co.

Keller, Helen. (2000). To Love this Life: Quotations from Helen Keller. American Foundation for the Blind.

Life Applications Study Bible. (1996). Tydale House Publishers, Wheaton, Illinois.

Mandela, Nelson. (1994). Nelson Mandela: The Struggle Is My Life: His Speeches and Writings Brought Together with Historical Documents and Accounts of Mandela in Prison by Fellow-Prisoners. Mayibuye Books.

Mandela, Nelson. (1994). A Time to Build: Addresses by the President, Mr. Nelson R. Mandela, at His Inauguration, the Opening of Parliament (May 1994) and at the OAU Meeting in Tunis (June 1994). South African Communication Service.

Navin, Chawla. (2002). Mother Theresa. Lightening Source Inc.

Schraff, Anne E. (2004). Wilma Rudolph: the Greatest Woman Sprinter in History. Enslow Pub Inc.

Schweitzer, Albert. (1995). Edited By: Richard Kik. The Light Within Us. Philosophical Library.

Schweitzer, Albert. (1996). The Spiritual Life Edited By: Charles R. Joy. The ECCO Press.

Tada, Joni Eareckson. (1997). When God Weeps: Why Our Sufferings Matter to the Almighty. Zondervan.Tada, Joni Eareckson. (2001). Joni: An Unforgettable Story. Zondervan.

Wines, Leslie. (2000). (ed). Rumi: A Spiritual Biography. Natl Book Network.

Ziedonis D, Berman J, Lehn MD, Colameco S. (2008) Support Groups and 12-Step Programs in the treatment of Chronic pain. In Pain and Chemical Dependency. (pp. 271-285) Smith HS (ed). Oxford University Press, USA

About the Author

Stephen Colameco, M.D., M.Ed. is an addiction specialist. He has served as a health system medical director, director of medical education, family medicine residency director and as a medical director providing chronic pain case management consulting services. In 2003, he was recognized for his contributions to his specialty as one of 219 fellows by the American Society of Addiction Medicine. Dr. Colameco lectures and has written journal articles about pain management and addiction. He strongly supports evidenced-based medical practice. As a believer in the value of mind-body medicine, he practices yoga and meditation.

More information about the Dr. Colameco can be found on his website—AddictionPain.com.

Made in the USA
San Bernardino, CA
21 December 2013